Mood and Anxiety Disorders During Pregnancy and Postpartum

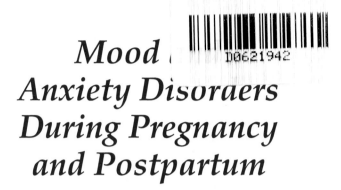

EDITED BY

Lee S. Cohen, M.D.
Ruta M. Nonacs, M.D., Ph.D.

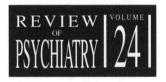

REVIEW OF PSYCHIATRY | VOLUME 24

No. 4

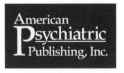

American Psychiatric Publishing, Inc.

Washington, DC
London, England

Manufactured in the United States of America on acid-free paper
09 08 07 06 05   5 4 3 2 1
First Edition

Typeset in Adobe's Palatino.

American Psychiatric Publishing, Inc.
1000 Wilson Boulevard
Arlington, VA 22209-3901
www.appi.org

The correct citation for this book is
Cohen, Lee S., Nonacs, Ruta M. (editors): *Mood and Anxiety Disorders During Pregnancy and Postpartum* (Review of Psychiatry Series, Volume 24, Number 4; Oldham JM and Riba MB, series editors). Washington, DC, American Psychiatric Publishing, 2005

Library of Congress Cataloging-in-Publication Data
Mood and anxiety disorders during pregnancy and postpartum / edited by
    Lee S. Cohen, Ruta M. Nonacs.—1st ed.
        p. ; cm.—(Review of psychiatry series ; v. 24, 4)
    Includes bibliographical references and index.
    ISBN 1-58562-225-7 (pbk. : alk. paper)
        1. Mental illness in pregnancy. 2. Postpartum depression. 3. Affective
    disorders. 4. Anxiety in women. I. Cohen, Lee S. II. Nonacs, Ruta. III. Series.
        [DNLM: 1. Anxiety Disorders—Pregnancy. 2. Mood Disorders—Pregnancy.
    3. Depression, Postpartum. 4. Postpartum Period—psychology. WQ 240 M817
    2005]
    RG588.M66 2005
    618.7′6—dc22

                                                                              2005004568

British Library Cataloguing in Publication Data
A CIP record is available from the British Library.

Mood and Anxiety Disorders During Pregnancy and Postpartum

Review of Psychiatry Series
John M. Oldham, M.D., M.S.
Michelle B. Riba, M.D., M.S.
Series Editors

Contents

Contributors

Ross J. Baldessarini, M.D.
Professor of Psychiatry (Neuroscience), Harvard Medical School, Boston, Massachusetts; Director, McLean Psychopharmacology Program, Neuropsychopharmacology Laboratory and International Consortium for Bipolar Disorder Research, McLean Hospital, Belmont, Massachusetts

Lee S. Cohen, M.D.
Associate Professor of Psychiatry, Harvard Medical School; Director, Perinatal and Reproductive Psychiatry Clinical Research Program, Clinical Psychopharmacology Unit, Department of Psychiatry, Massachusetts General Hospital, Boston, Massachusetts

Juliana Mogielnicki, B.A.
Perinatal and Reproductive Psychiatry Clinical Research Program, Clinical Psychopharmacology Unit, Department of Psychiatry, Massachusetts General Hospital, Boston, Massachusetts

D. Jeffrey Newport, M.D., M.S., M.Div.
Assistant Professor, Department of Psychiatry and Behavioral Sciences, Emory University School of Medicine, Atlanta, Georgia

Ruta M. Nonacs, M.D., Ph.D.
Instructor in Psychiatry, Harvard Medical School; Associate Director, Perinatal and Reproductive Psychiatry Clinical Research Program, Clinical Psychopharmacology Unit, Department of Psychiatry, Massachusetts General Hospital, Boston, Massachusetts

John M. Oldham, M.D., M.S.
Professor and Chair, Department of Psychiatry and Behavioral Sciences, Medical University of South Carolina, Charleston, South Carolina

Laura Fagioli Petrillo, M.D.
Instructor in Psychiatry, Harvard Medical School and Perinatal and Reproductive Psychiatry Clinical Research Program, Clinical Psychopharmacology Unit, Department of Psychiatry, Massachusetts General Hospital, Boston, Massachusetts

Kimberly Ragan, M.S.W.
LMSW, Department of Psychiatry and Behavioral Sciences, Emory University School of Medicine, Atlanta, Georgia

Michelle B. Riba, M.D., M.S.
Clinical Professor and Associate Chair for Education and Academic Affairs, Department of Psychiatry, University of Michigan Medical School, Ann Arbor, Michigan

Zachary N. Stowe, M.D.
Associate Professor, Departments of Psychiatry and Behavioral Sciences and Gynecology and Obstetrics, Emory University School of Medicine, Atlanta, Georgia

Adele C. Viguera, M.D.
Assistant Professor of Psychiatry, Harvard Medical School; Associate Director, Perinatal and Reproductive Psychiatry Clinical Research Program, Clinical Psychopharmacology Unit, Department of Psychiatry, Massachusetts General Hospital, Boston, Massachusetts

Introduction to the Review of Psychiatry Series

John M. Oldham, M.D., M.S.
Michelle B. Riba, M.D., M.S.

2005 REVIEW OF PSYCHIATRY SERIES TITLES

- *Psychiatric Genetics*
  EDITED BY KENNETH S. KENDLER, M.D., AND
  LINDON EAVES, PH.D., D.SC.

- *Sleep Disorders and Psychiatry*
  EDITED BY DANIEL J. BUYSSE, M.D.

- *Advances in Treatment of Bipolar Disorder*
  EDITED BY TERENCE A. KETTER, M.D.

- *Mood and Anxiety Disorders During Pregnancy and Postpartum*
  EDITED BY LEE S. COHEN, M.D., AND RUTA M. NONACS, M.D., PH.D.

The Annual Review of Psychiatry has been published for almost a quarter of a century, and 2005 marks the final year of publication of this highly successful series. First published in 1982, the Annual Review was conceived as a single volume highlighting new developments in the field that would be informative and of practical value to mental health practitioners. From the outset, the Annual Review was coordinated with the Annual Meeting of the American Psychiatric Association (APA), so that the material from each year's volume could also be presented in person by the chapter authors at the Annual Meeting. In its early years, the Review was one of a relatively small number of major books regularly published by American Psychiatric Press, Inc. (APPI; now American Psychiatric Publishing, Inc.). Through the subsequent years, however, the demand for new authoritative material led to an exponential growth in the number of new titles published by APPI each year. New published material became more readily available throughout each year, so that the unique function originally provided by the Annual Review was no longer needed.

Times change in many ways. The increased production volume, depth, and diversity of APPI's timely and authoritative material, now rapidly being augmented by electronic publishing, are welcome changes, and it is appropriate that this year's volume of the Annual Review represents the final curtain of the series. We have been privileged to be coeditors of the Annual Review for over a decade, and we are proud to have been a part of this distinguished series.

We hope you will agree that Volume 24 wonderfully lives up to the traditionally high standards of the Annual Review. In *Psychiatric Genetics,* edited by Kendler and Eaves, the fast-breaking and complex world of the genetics of psychiatric disorders is addressed. Following Kendler's clear and insightful introductory overview, Eaves, Chen, Neale, Maes, and Silberg present a careful analysis of the various methodologies used today to study the genetics of complex diseases in human populations. In turn, the book presents the latest findings on the genetics of schizophrenia, by Riley and Kendler; of anxiety disorders, by Hettema; of substance use disorders, by Prescott, Maes, and Kendler; and of antisocial behavior, by Jacobson.

Sleep Disorders and Psychiatry, edited by Buysse, brings us up to date on the sleep disorders from a psychiatric perspective, reviewing critically important clinical conditions that may not always receive the priority they deserve. Following a comprehensive introductory chapter, Buysse then presents, with his colleagues Germain, Moul, and Nofzinger, an authoritative review of the fundamental and pervasive problem of insomnia. Strollo and Davé next review sleep apnea, a potentially life-threatening condition that can also be an unrecognized source of excessive daytime sleepiness and impaired functioning. Black, Nishino, and Brooks present the basics of narcolepsy, along with new findings and treatment recommendations. In two separate chapters, Winkelman then reviews the parasomnias and the particular problem of restless legs syndrome. The book concludes with an extremely important chapter by Zee and Manthena reviewing circadian rhythm sleep disorders.

Advances in Treatment of Bipolar Disorder, edited by Ketter, provides an update on bipolar disorder. Following an introductory overview by Ketter, Sachs, Bowden, Calabrese, Chang, and Rasgon on the advances in the treatment of bipolar disorder, more specific material is presented on the treatment of acute mania, by Ketter, Wang, Nowakowska, Marsh, and Bonner. Sachs then presents a current look at the treatment of acute depression in bipolar patients, followed by a review by Bowden and Singh of the long-term management of bipolar disorder. The problem of rapid cycling is taken up by Muzina, Elhaj, Gajwani, Gao, and Calabrese. Chang, Howe, and Simeonova then discuss the treatment of children and adolescents with bipolar disorder, and the concluding chapter, by Rasgon and Zappert, provides a special focus on women with bipolar disorder.

Mood and Anxiety Disorders During Pregnancy and Postpartum, edited by Cohen and Nonacs, concerns the range of issues of psychiatric relevance related to pregnancy and the postpartum period. Cohen and Nonacs review the course of psychiatric illness during pregnancy, and the postpartum period is covered by Petrillo, Nonacs, Viguera, and Cohen. In this review, the authors focus particularly on depression, bipolar disorder, anxiety disorders, and psychotic disorders. The diagnosis and treatment of mood and anxiety disorders during pregnancy are then discussed in more detail in the subsequent chapter by Nonacs, Cohen, Viguera, and Mogielnicki, followed by a more in-depth look at management of bipolar disorder by Viguera, Cohen, Nonacs, and Baldessarini. Nonacs then presents a comprehensive and important look at the postpartum period, concentrating on mood disorders. This chapter is followed by a discussion of the use of antidepressants and mood-stabilizing medications during breast-feeding, by Ragan, Stowe, and Newport. Overall, this book provides up-to-date information about the management of common psychiatric disorders during gestation and during the critical postpartum period.

Before closing this final version of our annual introductory comments, we would like to thank all of the authors who have contributed so generously to the Annual Review, as well as the editors who preceded us. In addition, we thank the wonderful staff at APPI who have so diligently helped produce a quality product each year, and we would particularly like to thank our two administrative assistants, Liz Bednarowicz and Linda Gacioch, without whom the work could not have been done.

Preface

Lee S. Cohen, M.D.
Ruta M. Nonacs, M.D., Ph.D.

The last decade has brought growing interest in women's mental health. The number of original reports in the literature and academic symposia addressing issues in reproductive psychiatry has expanded dramatically. Nonetheless, data from systematic study of several critical areas in women's mental health lag behind the scope of clinical questions that patients raise in the context of their treatment. This is particularly the case as patients present for information regarding the course and treatment of psychiatric illness during pregnancy, the postpartum period, and lactation.

Mood and Anxiety Disorders During Pregnancy and Postpartum represents an effort to address a spectrum of critical areas that inform the clinical care of women during the childbearing years. Several chapters describe more recent studies which suggest that pregnancy is not "protective" with regard to risk for new onset or relapse of psychiatric illness. If pregnancy does not afford emotional well-being for women, then those who provide clinical care and advice to women during this important time must have the ability to weigh the risks of treating patients with a spectrum of therapies against the risks of deferring treatment and placing patients at risk for the effects of untreated psychiatric illness. Clinicians must also be familiar with the importance of screening and adequately treating postpartum depression, which, when untreated, is associated with significant morbidity for mother, child, and families.

Despite the numerous studies describing the substantial prevalence of depression in postpartum women, routine screening of the illness is uncommon, and the disorder remains typically untreated or incompletely managed. Many women decline or defer treatment of postpartum depression because of the impression that pharmacologic intervention during this time is incompatible with beast-feeding. However, research regarding the use of psychotropics during lactation over the last several years rivals information regarding the majority of other therapeutic and nonprescription compounds that women ingest while lactating.

Hopefully, this volume will help the clinician to collaborate with patients who have experienced or who are currently experiencing psychiatric illness but who wish to conceive, who are pregnant, or who are in the postpartum period. The chapters in this volume do not provide perfect answers to the difficult clinical situations faced by those who work with patients suffering from psychiatric illness during the childbearing years. But the reader will conclude that there are thoughtful ways to navigate these clinical courses and that such an approach can be achieved with patients in a collaborative fashion. Such a clinical approach minimizes the morbidity associated with untreated psychiatric illness during these critical times in the lives of women.

Chapter 1

Course of Psychiatric Illness During Pregnancy and the Postpartum

Laura Fagioli Petrillo, M.D.
Ruta M. Nonacs, M.D., Ph.D.
Adele C. Viguera, M.D.
Lee S. Cohen, M.D.

Although the postpartum period has been identified as a time of increased vulnerability to psychiatric illness, pregnancy has often been considered a time of emotional well-being for women (Zajicek 1981). However, studies now suggest that relapse of an existing psychiatric condition or the emergence of a new disorder is often seen during pregnancy (Cohen et al. 1994a, 1996; Evans et al. 2001; Frank et al. 1987; Northcott and Stein 1994; O'Hara 1986). Mood and anxiety disorders are highly prevalent among women of childbearing age (Eaton et al. 1994; Kessler et al. 1993), as is psychopharmacologic treatment for these disorders. Because of the limited amount of information regarding the use of psychotropic medications during pregnancy, many women are advised to discontinue such medications prior to attempts to conceive. Although some reports suggest that women remain well during pregnancy, many studies have demonstrated high rates of recurrent psychiatric illness in women who elect to discontinue maintenance treatment during pregnancy.

Growing evidence suggests that active maternal psychiatric illness during pregnancy and the postpartum period can negatively affect child development and can cause significant morbidity for the mother. Investigating the course and treatment of maternal psychiatric illness during these times is therefore a priority. Pharmacologic treatment of psychiatric disorders should involve a process of weighing the risks and benefits of proposed interventions and the documented (Orr and Miller 1995; Steer et al. 1992) and theoretical risks associated with untreated psychiatric disorders. In pregnancy, this process can become more difficult because of issues related to neonatal exposure to psychotropic agents. Therefore, the threshold for the pharmacologic treatment of psychiatric disorders tends to be higher during pregnancy than in other conditions. Typically, such treatment is reserved for situations in which the disorder interferes significantly with maternal and fetal well-being.

Despite the growing number of reviews on the subject, management of antenatal psychiatric illness is still largely guided by practical experience, with few definitive data and no controlled treatment studies to inform treatment. The most appropriate treatment algorithm depends on the severity of the disorder—and ultimately on the wishes of the patient. Clinicians must work collaboratively with the patient to arrive at the safest decision based on a constellation of factors, including her psychiatric history, current symptoms, and attitude toward the use of psychiatric medications during pregnancy. Information regarding the course of psychiatric illness during pregnancy and the postpartum period may also help to guide these decisions.

Unipolar Depression

Women are twice as likely as men to experience an affective disorder, and the peak incidence of these disorders occurs during the childbearing years, between the ages of 25 and 44 (Kessler et al. 1993). Early reports described pregnancy as a time of affective well-being that conferred "protection" against psychiatric illness (Kendell et al. 1976, 1987; Kumar and Robson 1984; Zajicek 1981). However, more recent studies have indicated that women remain at high risk for depression during pregnancy. At least one prospective study has described equal rates of major and minor depression (approximating 10%) in gravid and nongravid women (O'Hara et al. 1990). Several other studies have also noted high rates of clinically significant depressive symptoms during pregnancy (Gotlib et al. 1989; O'Hara 1986, 1995). Data from a large-scale cohort study of 14,000 women suggested that antenatal depressive symptoms may be more common than postpartum depression (Evans et al. 2001). A personal history of affective illness significantly increases the risk of antenatal depression (Gotlib et al. 1989; O'Hara 1995); however, for about one-third of the women who become depressed during pregnancy, this represents the first episode of major depression (O'Hara 1995). Other risk factors for antenatal depression include marital discord or dissatisfaction, inadequate psychosocial supports, recent adverse life events, lower socioeconomic status, and unwanted pregnancy (Gotlib et al. 1989; O'Hara 1986, 1995).

Women with recurrent major depression who have been maintained on an antidepressant medication prior to conception appear to be at especially high risk for relapse during pregnancy (Cohen et al. 2004a). Although there are accumulating data to support the relative safety of using certain antidepressants during pregnancy, women commonly choose or are counseled to discontinue antidepressant treatment during pregnancy. A large body of literature in nongravid populations indicates that the discontinuation of maintenance pharmacologic treatment is associated with high rates of relapse (Baldessarini and Tondo 1998; Kupfer et al. 1992; Viguera et al. 1998). Preliminary data suggest that pregnancy does not protect against relapse in the setting of medication discontinuation. In a recent prospective study of 32 women with recurrent major depression who discontinued antidepressant medication near the time of conception, approximately 75% relapsed during pregnancy, typically during the first trimester (Cohen et al. 2004a).

Although more severe forms of affective illness may be readily detected, depression that emerges during pregnancy is frequently overlooked. Many of the neurovegetative signs and symptoms characteristic of major depression (e.g., sleep and appetite disturbance, diminished libido, low energy) are also observed in nondepressed women during pregnancy. In addition, certain medical disorders commonly seen during pregnancy, such as anemia, gestational diabetes, and thyroid dysfunction, may be associated with depressive symptoms and may complicate the diagnosis of depression during pregnancy. Clinical features that may support the diagnosis of major depression include anhedonia, feelings of guilt and hopelessness, and suicidal thoughts. Suicidal ideation is often reported; however, risk of self-injurious or suicidal behaviors appears to be relatively low in the population of women who develop depression during pregnancy (Appleby 1991; O'Hara et al. 1984).

About 10%–15% of women experience depressive symptoms during the first 3 months after delivery (Kumar and Robson 1984; O'Hara et al. 1984). Women with histories of major depression are particularly vulnerable to illness during the postpartum period. Although studies carried out in the general population suggest a twofold increase in risk among women with a history of unipolar depression (O'Hara 1995), a recent prospective study of 47 women with recurrent major depressive disorder suggests that the risk of postpartum illness in women with this history may be as high as 50% (Nonacs et al. 2004).

Bipolar Disorder

The impact of pregnancy on the natural course of bipolar disorder is not well described. Although several studies suggest that pregnancy may have a protective effect with regard to risk of recurrent illness in women with bipolar disorder (Grof et al. 2000; Lier et al. 1989), other studies demonstrate high rates of relapse during pregnancy (Akdeniz et al. 2003; Viguera et al. 2002). In patients who discontinue mood stabilizers, the risk is even higher. In a recent retrospective study of 42 women with bipolar disorder who discontinued lithium maintenance treatment proximate to conception, 52.3% experienced recurrent symptoms during pregnancy (Viguera et al. 2000). In contrast, none of the 9 women who maintained lithium treatment during pregnancy relapsed.

Similarly, the risk for relapse of bipolar disorder during the postpartum period is high. One retrospective study examined recurrence rates during pregnancy and after delivery in 42 women with bipolar disorder, after the discontinuation of lithium maintenance, compared with recurrence rates in 59 age-matched non-pregnant women (Viguera et al. 2000). Although recurrence rates among the pregnant women were similar to those rates in the nonpregnant control subjects, recurrences of illness were 2.9 times more frequent in the postpartum compared with nonpregnant women. These findings suggest that risk of recurrent illness increases sharply during the postpartum period. In this study, 70% of women with bipolar disorder experienced illness during the postpartum period. Although those women who experienced recurrent symptoms during pregnancy were at highest risk for illness after delivery, recurrent illness occurred at high rates in women who were euthymic during pregnancy (Nonacs et al. 1999). None of the patients in this study developed psychotic symptoms; however, other studies have demonstrated that women with bipolar disorder are at high risk for developing postpartum psychosis (Dean et al. 1989; Reich and Winokur 1970).

Pregnancy in women with bipolar disorder should be considered a strong risk factor for relapse, whether or not the woman is taking a psychotropic medication. Accordingly, close monitoring of these patients is necessary during pregnancy and the postpartum period. Rapid intervention can significantly reduce morbidity and improve overall prognosis.

Anxiety Disorders

Although modest to moderate levels of anxiety during pregnancy are common, pathologic anxiety may occur in certain women. Anxiety disorders are common among women, but little is known about the prevalence of anxiety disorders during pregnancy and the postpartum period. In a recent prospective longitudinal study of a community sample of 8,323 pregnant women in England, it was observed that 21.9% of the women had clinically significant symptoms of anxiety (Heron et al. 2004). Among the women who reported elevated levels of anxiety during pregnancy, most (64%) also reported elevated levels of anxiety after delivery. Furthermore, antenatal anxiety predicted postpartum depression at 8 weeks and at 8 months, even after controlling for the presence of antenatal depression.

There are few data regarding the impact of pregnancy on the course of specific anxiety disorders. Several anecdotal reports and case series have described a reduction in the severity and frequency of panic symptoms during pregnancy (Cowley and Roy-Byrne 1989; George et al. 1987; Klein et al. 1994–1995; Villeponteaux et al. 1992). For example, in a retrospective study of 20 women with a total of 33 pregnancies, the majority of women reported a marked symptomatic improvement during pregnancy (Klein et al. 1994–1995). Other authors have observed that some patients were able to discontinue antipanic medications during pregnancy without relapse of their panic disorder (George et al. 1987; Villeponteaux et al. 1992). Other studies, however, have noted the persistence or worsening of panic-related symptoms during pregnancy (see Cohen et al. 1994a, 1994b, 2004b; Northcott and Stein 1994). In a recent prospective study of 36 women with pregravid histories of panic disorder, 44% experienced recurrent panic symptoms during pregnancy (Cohen et al. 2004b). Women who discontinued antipanic treatment were three times as likely to relapse during pregnancy as were those who maintained treatment.

Although the course of panic during pregnancy is variable, the postpartum period appears to be a time of increased vulnerability to panic symptoms (Cohen et al. 1994b, 1996; Cowley and Roy-Byrne 1989; George et al. 1987; Northcott and Stein 1994). Several studies also describe the first onset of panic disorder during the puerperium (Metz et al. 1988; Sholomskas et al. 1993; Wisner et al. 1996). Sholomskas and colleagues (1993) reported the first lifetime onset of panic disorder during the postpartum period in 10.9% of the 64 women with panic disorder studied, a significantly higher rate than expected for a given 12-week period. This finding suggests that the emergence of panic disorder in the puerperium is not simply coincidental.

Among women with pregravid histories of panic disorder, a significant increase in the severity or frequency of attacks during the postpartum period appears to be a consistent finding, occurring in 31%–63% of women after delivery (Cohen et al. 1994b; Northcott and Stein 1994). Postpartum exacerbation occurs commonly even in those women who were symptom-free during pregnancy (Wisner et al. 1996). In one study, those patients who received antipanic pharmacotherapy during the third trimester were less likely to develop puerperal worsening of panic symptoms (Cohen et al. 1994b).

The course of obsessive-compulsive disorder (OCD) during pregnancy has not been studied systematically. It appears that some women may have the first onset of OCD symptoms during pregnancy (Buttolph and Holland 1990). Several studies indicate that women may even be at increased risk for the onset of OCD during pregnancy and the puerperium period (Buttolph and Holland 1990; Maina et al. 1999; Neziroglu et al. 1992; Sichel et al. 1993a).

In women with pregravid histories of OCD, retrospective studies have shown that pregnancy may precipitate a worsening of symptoms in some (Buttolph and Holland 1990; Neziroglu et al. 1992; Williams and Koran 1997). Buttolph and Holland (1990) reported that 27 (69%) of 39 women reported the onset or worsening of OCD symptoms during pregnancy. This group of women is at high risk for relapse in the setting of medication discontinuation. In one prospectively studied group of patients with OCD, 43% relapsed during pregnancy in the context of medication discontinuation (Sichel et al. 1993a).

Retrospective studies also indicate that some women may experience acute onset of OCD within the first few weeks after giving birth (Buttolph and Holland 1990; Sichel et al. 1993b). The most common features in "postpartum OCD" are intrusive, egodystonic, obsessional thoughts about harming the newborn infant and avoidance of situations that evoke these kinds of cognitions. In women with pregravid histories of OCD, the postpartum period is a time of risk. Women with pregravid histories of OCD may also be at increased risk for developing postpartum depression (Abramowitz et al. 2003).

Posttraumatic stress disorder (PTSD) is twice as prevalent in women as in men (Kessler et al. 1995). Given its high prevalence among women, its course in pregnancy has been surprisingly understudied, and many of the data have their basis in case reports. PTSD has been described during pregnancy in cases where the woman experienced a complicated prior delivery (Ballard et al.

1995). PTSD may also present during the postpartum period; prolonged labor, severe pain during childbirth, and feeling a loss of control during delivery appear to be risk factors (Ballard et al. 1995). Postpartum PTSD may affect a woman's decisions about future childbearing, may decrease her ability to breast-feed, and may impair parent-child bonding (Reynolds 1997). Thus, significant morbidity exists during the postpartum period and may affect future pregnancies for women who have had traumatic birth experiences, making close monitoring of these women during and after pregnancy essential.

Psychotic Disorders

Although anecdotal reports and one epidemiologic study (Spielvogel and Wile 1992; Wrede et al. 1980) describe improvement of symptoms in some women with chronic psychotic illnesses during pregnancy, the data suggest that maternal and neonatal morbidity associated with such illness are significant. Studies show that women with chronic psychotic disorders are at increased risk for poor fetal outcome, including stillbirth, preterm delivery, low birth weight, and infant death (Spielvogel and Wile 1992; Wrede et al. 1980). Another study did not confirm an increased risk of obstetric complications (Wrede et al. 1980). Maternal tobacco, alcohol, and drug use and low socioeconomic status are potential contributors to the negative outcomes observed (Spielvogel and Wile 1992; Wrede et al. 1980).

Acute psychosis during pregnancy is both an obstetric and a psychiatric emergency. Similar to other psychiatric symptoms of new onset, first onset of psychosis during pregnancy cannot be presumed to be reactive; it requires a systematic diagnostic evaluation. Psychosis during pregnancy may inhibit a woman's ability to obtain appropriate and necessary prenatal care and may impede her ability to cooperate with caregivers during delivery (Miller 1990; Spielvogel and Wile 1992; Wrede et al. 1980). Furthermore, case reports of psychosis during pregnancy suggest that it increases the risk of postpartum psychosis (Spielvogel and Wile 1992; Wrede et al. 1980).

Risks of Untreated Illness in the Mother

Although clinicians have appropriate concern regarding the risks associated with fetal exposure to psychiatric medications, the potential impact of untreated psychiatric illness on the child's well-being has often been overlooked. Depression may be associated with significant morbidity in the mother. It increases the risk of self-injurious or suicidal behaviors in the mother but also may contribute to inadequate self-care and poor compliance with prenatal care. Women with depression often present with decreased appetite and consequently lower-than-expected weight gain in pregnancy, factors that may be associated with negative pregnancy outcomes (Zuckerman et al. 1989). In addition, pregnant women with depression are more likely to smoke and to use either alcohol or illicit drugs, behaviors that further increase risk to the fetus (Zuckerman et al. 1989).

In addition, maternal depression itself may adversely affect the developing fetus. Although it has been difficult to assess the impact of antenatal depression on fetal development and neonatal well-being in humans, several studies have found an association between maternal depression and factors that predict poor neonatal outcome, including preterm birth, lower birth weight, smaller head circumference, and lower Apgar scores for physical condition of the neonate (Dayan et al. 2002; Orr and Miller 1995; Orr et al. 2002; Steer et al. 1992; Zuckerman et al. 1990).

Anxiety symptoms have also been associated with poor neonatal outcome and obstetric complications, including low Apgar scores, premature labor, and low birth weight (Cohen et al. 1989; Crandon 1979; Istvan 1986). Additionally, antenatal anxiety has been linked to childhood behavioral problems (O'Connor et al. 2003). Furthermore, one prospective, longitudinal study of 8,323 women suggested that antenatal anxiety predicts postpartum anxiety and depression (Heron et al. 2004). This is concerning because maternal mood disturbances postpartum may negatively affect childhood development (Murray 1992; Murray and Cooper 1996).

The physiologic mechanisms by which symptoms of depression and anxiety might affect neonatal outcome are not clear. However, increased serum cortisol and catecholamine levels, which are typically observed in patients with depression and anxiety, may affect placental function by altering uterine blood flow and inducing uterine irritability (Glover 1997; Teixeira et al. 1999). Dysregulation of the hypothalamic-pituitary-adrenal (HPA) axis that is associated with depression may also have a direct effect on fetal development. Animal studies suggest that stress during pregnancy is also associated with neuronal death and abnormal development of neural structures in the fetal brain, as well as sustained dysfunction on the HPA axis in the offspring (see Alves et al. 1997; Glover 1997).

Maternal depression and other types of psychiatric illness may also have a significant impact on the family unit. Depression is typically associated with interpersonal difficulties, and disruptions in mother-child interactions and attachment may have a profound impact on infant development. Recent research indicates that children of depressed mothers are more likely to have behavioral problems and to exhibit disruptions in cognitive and emotional development (Murray 1992; Viguera et al. 1997; Weinberg and Tronick 1998). Furthermore, depression during pregnancy significantly increases a woman's risk for developing postpartum depression (Gotlib et al. 1989; O'Hara et al. 1984). Thus, antenatal depression may have significant negative effects that extend well beyond the pregnancy.

Conclusion

Pregnancy previously had been considered protective with respect to the risk for psychiatric illness, but emerging data contradict that belief. Psychiatric disorders may have their initial presentation during pregnancy; more often, however, clinical presentations represent persistence or exacerbation of an already existing illness. Physicians therefore should screen aggressively for psychiatric disorders either prior to conception or during pregnancy, integrating questions about psychiatric symptoms and treatment into the obstetric history. Identification of women at risk and awareness of the data describing the course of psychiatric illness during pregnancy allow for the most thoughtful acute treatment before, during, and after pregnancy and afford opportunities for use of prophylactic strategies in order to prevent psychiatric disturbances in women during the childbearing years.

References

Abramowitz JS, Schwartz SA, Moore KM, et al: Obsessive-compulsive symptoms in pregnancy and the puerperium: a review of the literature. J Anxiety Disord 17:461–478, 2003

Akdeniz F, Vahip S, Pirildar S, et al: Risk factors associated with childbearing-related episodes in women with bipolar disorder. Psychopathology 36:234–238, 2003

Alves SE, Akbari HM, Anderson GM, et al: Neonatal ACTH administration elicits long-term changes in forebrain monoamine innervation: subsequent disruptions in hypothalamic-pituitary-adrenal and gonadal function. Ann NY Acad Sci 814:226–251, 1997

Appleby L: Suicide during pregnancy and in the first postnatal year. BMJ 302:137–140, 1991

Baldessarini R, Tondo L: Effects of lithium treatment in bipolar disorders and post-treatment-discontinuation reoccurrence risk. Clinical Drug Investigation 15:337–351, 1998

Ballard CG, Stanley AK, Brockington IF: Post-traumatic stress disorder (PTSD) after childbirth. Br J Psychiatry 166:525–528, 1995

Buttolph ML, Holland A: Obsessive compulsive disorders in pregnancy and childbirth, in Obsessive-Compulsive Disorders: Theory and Management. Edited by Jenike MA, Baer L, Minichiello WE. Chicago, IL, Year Book Medical, 1990, pp 89–97

Cohen LS, Rosenbaum JF, Heller VL: Panic attack–associated placental abruption: a case report. J Clin Psychiatry 50:266–267, 1989

Cohen LS, Sichel DA, Dimmock JA, et al: Impact of pregnancy on panic disorder: a case series. J Clin Psychiatry 55:284–288, 1994a

Cohen LS, Sichel DA, Dimmock JA, et al: Postpartum course in women with preexisting panic disorder. J Clin Psychiatry 55:289–292, 1994b

Cohen LS, Sichel DA, Faraone SV, et al: Course of panic disorder during pregnancy and the puerperium: a preliminary study. Biol Psychiatry 39:950–954, 1996

Cohen LS, Nonacs RM, Bailey JW, et al: Relapse of depression during pregnancy following antidepressant discontinuation: a preliminary prospective study. Arch Women Ment Health 7:217–221, 2004a

Cohen L, Soares C, Otto M, et al: Relapse of panic disorder during pregnancy among patients who discontinue or maintain anti-panic medication: a preliminary prospective study. Presentation at the 157th annual meeting of the American Psychiatric Association, New York, NY, May 2004b

Cowley DS, Roy-Byrne PP: Panic disorder during pregnancy. J Psychosom Obstet Gynaecol 10:193–210, 1989

Crandon AJ: Maternal anxiety and neonatal wellbeing. J Psychosom Res 23:113–115, 1979

Dayan J, Creveuil C, Herlicoviez M, et al: Role of anxiety and depression in the onset of spontaneous preterm labor. Am J Epidemiol 155: 293–301, 2002

Dean C, Williams RJ, Brockington IF: Is puerperal psychosis the same as bipolar manic-depressive disorder? A family study. Psychol Med 19:637–647, 1989

Eaton WW, Kessler RC, Wittchen H-U, et al: Panic and panic disorder in the United States. Am J Psychiatry 151:413–420, 1994

Evans J, Heron J, Francomb H, et al: Cohort study of depressed mood during pregnancy and after childbirth. BMJ 323:257–260, 2001

Frank E, Kupfer DJ, Jacob M, et al: Pregnancy-related affective episodes among women with recurrent depression. Am J Psychiatry 144:288–293, 1987

George DT, Ladenheim JA, Nutt DJ: Effect of pregnancy on panic attacks. Am J Psychiatry 144:1078–1079, 1987

Glover V: Maternal stress or anxiety in pregnancy and emotional development of the child. Br J Psychiatry 171:105–106, 1997

Gotlib IH, Whiffen VE, Mount JH, et al: Prevalence rates and demographic characteristics associated with depression in pregnancy and the postpartum period. J Consult Clin Psychol 57:269–274, 1989

Grof P, Robbins W, Alda M, et al: Protective effect of pregnancy in women with lithium-responsive bipolar disorder. J Affect Disord 61:31–39, 2000

Heron J, O'Connor TG, Evans J, et al: The course of anxiety and depression through pregnancy and the postpartum in a community sample. J Affect Disord 80:65–73, 2004

Istvan J: Stress, anxiety, and birth outcome: a critical review of the evidence. Psychol Bull 100:331–348, 1986

Kendell RE, Wainwright S, Hailey A, et al: The influence of childbirth on psychiatric morbidity. Psychol Med 6:297–302, 1976

Kendell RE, Chalmers JC, Platz C: Epidemiology of puerperal psychoses. Br J Psychiatry 150:662–673, 1987

Kessler RC, McGonagle KA, Swartz M, et al: Sex and depression in the National Comorbidity Survey, I: lifetime prevalence, chronicity and recurrence. J Affect Disord 29:85–96, 1993

Kessler RC, Sonnega A, Bromet E, et al: Posttraumatic stress disorder in the National Comorbidity Survey. Arch Gen Psychiatry 52:1048–1060, 1995

Klein DF, Skrobala AM, Garfinkel DS: Preliminary look at the effects of pregnancy on the course of panic disorder. Anxiety 1:227–232, 1994–1995

Kumar R, Robson KM: A prospective study of emotional disorders in childbearing women. Br J Psychiatry 144:35–47, 1984

Kupfer D, Frank E, Perel J, et al: Five-year outcome for maintenance therapies in recurrent depression. Arch Gen Psychiatry 49:769–773, 1992

Lier L, Kastrup M, Rafaelsen O: Psychiatric illness in relation to pregnancy and childbirth, II: diagnostic profiles, psychosocial and perinatal aspects. Nord Psykiatr Tidsskr 43:535–542, 1989

Maina G, Albert U, Bogetto F, et al: Recent life events and obsessive-compulsive disorder (OCD): the role of pregnancy/delivery. Psychiatry Res 89:49–58, 1999

Metz A, Sichel DA, Goff DC: Postpartum panic disorder. J Clin Psychiatry 49:278–279, 1988

Miller LJ: Psychotic denial of pregnancy: phenomenology and clinical management. Hosp Community Psychiatry 41:1233–1237, 1990

Murray L: The impact of postnatal depression on infant development. J Child Psychol Psychiatry 33:543–561, 1992

Murray L, Cooper PJ: The impact of postpartum depression on child development. Int Rev Psychiatry 8:55–63, 1996

Neziroglu F, Anemone R, Yaryura-Tobias JA: Onset of obsessive-compulsive disorder in pregnancy. Am J Psychiatry 149:947–950, 1992

Nonacs R, Viguera A, Cohen L: Postpartum course of bipolar illness. Presentation at the 152nd annual meeting of the American Psychiatric Association, Washington, DC, May 1999

Nonacs R, Viguera A, Cohen L, et al: Risk for recurrent depression during the postpartum period: a prospective study. Presentation at the 157th annual meeting of the American Psychiatric Association, New York City, May 2004

Northcott CJ, Stein MB: Panic disorder in pregnancy. J Clin Psychiatry 55:539–542, 1994

O'Connor TG, Heron J, Golding J, et al: Maternal antenatal anxiety and behavioural/emotional problems in children: a test of a programming hypothesis. J Child Psychol Psychiatry 44:1025–1036, 2003

O'Hara MW: Social support, life events, and depression during pregnancy and the puerperium. Arch Gen Psychiatry 43:569–573, 1986

O'Hara MW: Postpartum Depression: Causes and Consequences. New York, Springer-Verlag, 1995

O'Hara MW, Neunaber DJ, Zekoski EM: Prospective study of postpartum depression: prevalence, course, and predictive factors. J Abnorm Psychol 93:158–171, 1984

O'Hara MW, Zekoski EM, Philipps LH, et al: Controlled prospective study of postpartum mood disorders: comparison of childbearing and nonchildbearing women. J Abnorm Psychol 99:3–15, 1990

Orr S, Miller C: Maternal depressive symptoms and the risk of poor pregnancy outcome: review of the literature and preliminary findings. Epidemiol Rev 17:165–171, 1995

Orr S, James SA, Blackmore Prince C: Maternal prenatal depressive symptoms and spontaneous preterm births among African-American women in Baltimore, Maryland. Am J Epidemiol 156:797–802, 2002

Reich T, Winokur G: Postpartum psychosis in patients with manic depressive disease. J Nerv Ment Dis 151:60–68, 1970

Reynolds JL: Post-traumatic stress disorder after childbirth: the phenomenon of traumatic birth. CMAJ 156:831–835, 1997

Sholomskas DE, Wickamaratne PJ, Dogolo L, et al: Postpartum onset of panic disorder: a coincidental event? J Clin Psychiatry 54:476–480, 1993

Sichel DA, Cohen LS, Dimmock JA, et al: Postpartum obsessive compulsive disorder: a case series. J Clin Psychiatry 54:156–159, 1993a

Sichel DA, Cohen LS, Rosenbaum JF, et al: Postpartum onset of obsessive-compulsive disorder. Psychosomatics 34:277–279, 1993b

Spielvogel A, Wile J: Treatment and outcomes of psychotic patients during pregnancy and childbirth. Birth 19:131–137, 1992

Steer RA, Scholl TO, Hediger ML, et al: Self-reported depression and negative pregnancy outcomes. J Clin Epidemiol 45:1093–1099, 1992

Teixeira JM, Fisk NM, Glover V: Association between maternal anxiety in pregnancy and increased uterine artery resistance index: cohort based study. BMJ 318:153–157, 1999

Viguera AC, Nonacs RM, Baldessarini RJ, et al: Relapse following discontinuation of lithium maintenance in pregnant women with bipolar disorder. Presentation at the 150th annual meeting of the American Psychiatric Association, San Diego, CA, May 17–22, 1997

Viguera AC, Baldessarini RJ, Friedberg J: Discontinuing antidepressant treatment in major depression. Harv Rev Psychiatry 5:293–306, 1998

Viguera AC, Nonacs RM, Cohen LS, et al: Risk of recurrence of bipolar disorder in pregnant and nonpregnant women after discontinuing lithium maintenance. Am J Psychiatry 157:179–184, 2000

Viguera AC, Cohen LS, Baldessarini RJ, et al: Managing bipolar disorder during pregnancy: weighing the risks and benefits. Can J Psychiatry 47:426–436, 2002

Villeponteaux VA, Lydiard RB, Laraia MT, et al: The effects of pregnancy on pre-existing panic disorder. J Clin Psychiatry 53:201–203, 1992

Weinberg M, Tronick E: The impact of maternal psychiatric illness on infant development. J Clin Psychiatry 59 (suppl 2):53–61, 1998

Williams K, Koran L: Obsessive-compulsive disorder in pregnancy, the puerperium, and the premenstruum. J Clin Psychiatry 58:330–334, 1997

Wisner KL, Peindl KS, Hanusa BH: Effects of childbearing on the natural history of panic disorder with comorbid mood disorder. J Affect Disord 41:173–180, 1996

Wrede G, Mednick S, Huttenen M: Pregnancy and delivery complications in the births of unselected series of Finnish children with schizophrenic mothers. Acta Psychiatr Scand 62:369–381, 1980

Zajicek E: Psychiatric problems during pregnancy, in Pregnancy: A Psychological and Social Study. Edited by Wolkind S, Zajicek E. London, Academic Press, 1981, pp 57–73

Zuckerman BS, Amaro H, Bauchner H, et al: Depression during pregnancy: relationship to prior health behaviors. Am J Obstet Gynecol 160:1107–1111, 1989

Zuckerman BS, Bauchner H, Parker S, et al: Maternal depressive symptoms during pregnancy, and newborn irritability. J Dev Behav Pediatr 11:190–194, 1990

Chapter 2

Diagnosis and Treatment of Mood and Anxiety Disorders in Pregnancy

Ruta M. Nonacs, M.D., Ph.D.
Lee S. Cohen, M.D.
Adele C. Viguera, M.D.
Juliana Mogielnicki, B.A.

Mood and anxiety disorders are common in women and typically emerge during the childbearing years (Kessler et al. 1993). With the availability of effective and well-tolerated pharmacologic treatments for psychiatric disorders, a growing number of women are treated with psychotropic medications during their reproductive years. While pregnancy has traditionally been considered a time of emotional well-being, recent data indicate that about 10% of women experience clinically significant depressive symptoms during pregnancy (antenatal depression) (Evans et al. 2001; Gotlib et al. 1989; O'Hara 1986, 1995). Furthermore, women with histories of mood and anxiety disorders appear to be at high risk for recurrent illness during pregnancy, particularly after medication is discontinued prior to pregnancy (Altshuler et al. 2001; Cohen et al. 2004a, 2004b).

Frequently, women with histories of psychiatric illness seek consultation regarding the potential risks associated with use of psychotropic medications during pregnancy, either prior to conception or early in the course of pregnancy. In other cases, women present with new onset or recurrence of symptoms during pregnancy. In both of these settings, the clinician faces certain challenges when making recommendations regarding the treatment of psychiatric illness during pregnancy. All medications diffuse readily across the placenta, and no psychotropic drug has yet been approved by the U.S. Food and Drug Administration (FDA) for use during pregnancy. Although data accumulated over the past 30 years suggest that some medications may be used safely during pregnancy (Altshuler et al. 1996; Cohen and Altshuler 1997; Wisner et al. 1999), knowledge regarding the risks of prenatal exposure to psychotropic medications is still incomplete. Thus, it is common for patients to avoid pharmacologic treatment during pregnancy. With increasing evidence of high rates of relapse following discontinuation of psychotropic agents, including antidepressants (Einarson et al. 2001b; Kupfer et al. 1992; Viguera et al. 1998), mood stabilizers (Suppes et al. 1991), antipsychotics (Dencker et al. 1986; Gitlin et al. 2001; Viguera et al. 1997), and benzodiazepines (Roy-Byrne et al. 1989), and given the high rates of psychiatric illness during pregnancy and the postpartum period (Evans et al. 2001; O'Hara 1986; O'Hara et al. 1991), the importance of psychiatric consultation in this setting is intuitive.

The clinical challenge for physicians who care for women with psychiatric disorders during pregnancy is to minimize risk to the fetus while limiting morbidity from untreated psychiatric illness in the mother. In contrast to many other clinical conditions for which treatment is maintained throughout the pregnancy, treatment of psychiatric disorders during pregnancy is typically reserved for situations in which the disorder interferes significantly with maternal well-being; thus, the threshold for the treatment of psychiatric disorders during pregnancy tends to be higher than the threshold for many other nonpsychiatric medical conditions. Because no decision is absolutely free of risk, it is imperative that clinical decisions regarding psychotropic drug use be made collaboratively with patients and their partners on a case-by-case basis. Physicians must provide accurate and current information on the reproductive safety of pharmacologic treatment and must help patients select the most appropriate treatment strategy. Even when given comparable information, patients may make different decisions regarding the use of pharmacologic therapy during pregnancy.

In this chapter, we review the available reproductive safety data regarding many agents used to treat mood and anxiety disorders during pregnancy. We then provide a conceptual framework that can be used for choosing appropriate pharmacotherapy for gravid women.

Prevalence of Mood and Anxiety Disorders During Pregnancy

Although some reports describe pregnancy as a time of affective well-being during which "protection" against psychiatric disorders is conferred, at least one prospective study describes equal rates of minor and major depression (approximating 10%) among gravid and nongravid women (O'Hara et al. 1990). Several other studies also note high rates (up to 20%) of clinically significant depressive symptoms during pregnancy (Evans et al. 2001; Gotlib et al. 1989; Marcus et al. 2003; O'Hara 1986, 1995). A personal history of affective illness significantly increases this risk (Gotlib et al. 1989; O'Hara 1995), and the risk appears to be particularly high among women with recurrent depression who discontinue maintenance treatment proximate to conception. A recent prospective study indicated that 75% of women who discontinue medication experience recurrent illness during pregnancy (Cohen et al. 2004a); in most cases, relapse occurred during the first trimester. Other risk factors for antenatal depression include marital discord or dissatisfaction, inadequate psychosocial supports, recent adverse life events, lower socioeconomic status, and unwanted pregnancy (Gotlib et al. 1989; O'Hara 1986, 1995).

Whereas certain psychiatric disorders may be readily detected during pregnancy (e.g., psychosis, panic disorder), depression that emerges during pregnancy is frequently overlooked. Many of the neurovegetative signs and symptoms characteristic of major and subsyndromal depression (e.g., disturbance in sleep and appetite, diminished libido, fatigue) are also observed in nondepressed women during pregnancy. In addition, certain medical disorders commonly seen during pregnancy, such as anemia, gestational diabetes, and thyroid dysfunction, may be associated with depressive symptoms and may complicate the diagnosis of depression during pregnancy (Klein and Essex 1995). Clinical features that may support the diagnosis of major depression during pregnancy include anhedonia, feelings of guilt and hopelessness, and suicidal thoughts. Suicidal ideation is not uncommon among depressed pregnant women; however, risk of self-injurious or suicidal behaviors appears to be relatively low in women who develop depression during pregnancy (Appleby 1991; Frautschi et al. 1994; Marzuk et al. 1997).

Although modest to moderate levels of anxiety during pregnancy are common, pathologic anxiety during pregnancy does occur and has been associated with poor neonatal outcome and obstetric complications (Andersson et al. 2004; Cohen et al. 1989; Crandon 1979; Istvan 1986). The prevalence of clinically significant anxiety symptoms during pregnancy has not been well studied. In a community sample of 8,323 pregnant women, it was observed that 21.9% of the women had clinically significant symptoms of anxiety (Heron et al. 2004). Although some reports suggest that women with pregravid histories of anxiety disorder may experience improvement in their symptoms during pregnancy, other studies report recurrent symptoms in women with pregravid histories of panic disorder and obsessive-compulsive disorder (OCD) (Cohen et al. 1994a, 1994b, 1996, 2004b; Northcott and Stein 1994). Rates of recurrent illness appear to be particularly high in women who discontinue pharmacologic treatment with anti-anxiety medications during pregnancy (Cohen et al. 2004a).

Risks of Untreated Maternal Illness During Pregnancy

While clinicians have appropriate concern regarding the known and unknown risks associated with fetal exposure to psychiatric medications, the potential impact of untreated psychiatric illness on maternal and fetal well-being has frequently been overlooked. Depression increases the risk of self-injurious or suicidal behaviors in the mother but also may contribute to inadequate self-care, including poor compliance with prenatal care. Women with depression or severe anxiety often present with decreased appetite and consequently lower-than-expected weight gain in pregnancy, factors that have been associated with negative pregnancy outcomes (Zuckerman et al. 1989). In addition, pregnant women with psychiatric illness are more likely to smoke and to use either alcohol or illicit drugs (Zuckerman et al. 1989)—behaviors that further increase risk to the fetus.

Current research suggests that maternal depression itself may adversely affect the developing fetus. Although it has been difficult to assess the impact of antenatal depression on fetal development and neonatal well-being in humans, several studies have found an association between maternal depression and factors that predict poor neonatal outcome, including preterm birth, lower birth-weight, smaller head circumference, and lower Apgar scores (Dayan et al. 2002; Orr and Miller 1995; Orr et al. 2002; Steer et al. 1992; Zuckerman et al. 1990).

Similarly, stress and anxiety during pregnancy have been associated with a variety of poor outcomes, including low Apgar scores, premature labor, low birth-weight, and placental abruption (Cohen et al. 1989; Crandon 1979; Istvan 1986). Additionally, antenatal anxiety has been linked to childhood behavioral problems (O'Connor et al. 2003). Furthermore, one recent prospective, longitudinal study of 8,323 women suggests that antenatal anxiety can predict postpartum anxiety and depression (Heron et al. 2004). This finding is concerning because postpartum mood disturbances may negatively impact childhood development.

The physiologic mechanisms by which symptoms of depression and anxiety might affect neonatal outcome are not clear. However, increased serum cortisol and catecholamine levels, typically observed in patients with anxiety and depression, may affect placental function by altering uterine blood flow and inducing uterine irritability (Glover 1997; Teixeira et al. 1999). Dysregulation of the hypothalamic-pituitary-adrenal (HPA) axis associated with depression and anxiety may also have a direct effect on fetal development. Animal studies suggest that stress during pregnancy is also associated with neuronal death and abnormal development of neural structures in fetal brain, as well as sustained dysfunction on the HPA axis in the offspring (Alves et al. 1997; Glover 1997).

Maternal depression may also have a significant impact on the family unit. Depression is typically associated with interpersonal difficulties, and disruptions in mother-child interactions and attachment may have a profound impact on infant development. Recent research indicates that children of depressed mothers are more likely to have behavioral problems and to exhibit disruptions in cognitive and emotional development (Murray 1992, 1997; Weinberg and Tronick 1998). Furthermore, depression during pregnancy significantly increases a woman's risk for developing postpartum depression (Gotlib et al. 1989; O'Hara et al. 1984). Summarily, antenatal depression may have significant adverse effects that extend well beyond pregnancy.

Treatment of Mood Disorders During Pregnancy

Weighing Treatment Options

With the advent of newer and better-tolerated antidepressants, as well as enhanced public awareness of available pharmacotherapy for depression, a growing number of women are prescribed antidepressant medications during the childbearing years. For women with recurrent major depression who are receiving maintenance antidepressant treatment and who plan to conceive, the clinician and patient must decide whether to maintain or to discontinue antidepressant treatment during pregnancy. Ideally, decisions regarding the use of psychotropic medications during pregnancy should be made prior to conception. Prior to pregnancy, the clinician must provide information regarding the patient's risk of relapse in the setting of medication discontinuation. The clinician must also take into account the risk of chronic, recurrent depression and its attendant morbidity in patients who experience depressive relapse after medication discontinuation (Keller et al. 1983; Mueller et al. 1999; Post 1992).

In patients with less severe depression, it may be appropriate to consider discontinuation of pharmacologic therapy during pregnancy. Nonpharmacologic interventions, including interpersonal psychotherapy (IPT) and cognitive-behavioral therapy (CBT), may be used prior to conception to facilitate the gradual tapering and discontinuation of an antidepressant medication in women planning to become pregnant. These modalities of treatment may reduce the risk of recurrent depressive symptoms during pregnancy, although this has not been studied systematically. Close monitoring during pregnancy is essential, even if all medications are discontinued and there is no apparent need for medication management. Women with histories of mood disorder who discontinue antidepressant treatment are at high risk for relapse, and early detection and treatment of recurrent illness during pregnancy may attenuate the morbidity associated with antenatal mood disorder.

Many women who discontinue antidepressant treatment during pregnancy do experience recurrent depressive symptoms. Thus, for women with more recurrent or refractory depressive illness, patient and clinician together may decide that the safest option that enhances the likelihood of sustaining euthymia is to continue pharmacologic treatment across pregnancy. In such a situation, the clinician should, when possible, select medications for use during pregnancy that have a well-characterized reproductive safety profile. Often this may involve switching from one psychotropic agent to another with a more complete reproductive safety profile. An example of this approach would be switching from mirtazapine, a medication for which there are almost no data regarding reproductive safety, to a better-characterized agent such as fluoxetine. In other situations, one may decide to use a medication for which information regarding reproductive safety is sparse. A example of such a scenario is when the clinician is treating refractory depressive illness in a patient who has been responsive to only one antidepressant and the data on reproductive safety are limited for that antidepressant (i.e., nefazodone). Such a patient may choose to continue this medication during pregnancy rather than risk relapse associated with discontinuation of the agent or a switch to another antidepressant.

Women may also experience new onset of depressive symptoms during pregnancy. For women who present with minor depressive symptoms, nonpharmacologic treatment strategies should be explored first. IPT or CBT may be beneficial for reducing the severity of depressive symptoms and may either limit or obviate the need for medications (Beck et al. 1979; Klerman et al. 1984; Spinelli 1997). In general, pharmacologic treatment is pursued when non-pharmacologic strategies have failed or when it is felt that the risks associated with psychiatric illness during pregnancy outweigh the risks of fetal exposure to a particular medication.

Nonpharmacologic Interventions

Until recently, there were few data on the role of nonpharmacologic treatments for depression during pregnancy. For women with mild to moderate depressive symptoms, nonpharmacologic interventions, including IPT (Klerman et al. 1984), cognitive therapy and CBT (Beck et al. 1979), and supportive psychotherapy, may be attractive alternatives to medication during pregnancy. In women who are receiving maintenance antidepressant treatment, non-pharmacologic interventions may potentially facilitate tapering of medication or may allow for use of lower dosages of medication.

IPT is a short-term, manual-driven psychotherapy that deals primarily with four major problem areas: grief, interpersonal disputes, role transitions, and interpersonal deficits (Keller et al. 1984). Given the importance of interpersonal relationships in couples expecting a child and the significant role transitions that take place during pregnancy and subsequent to delivery, IPT is ideally suited for the treatment of depressed pregnant women. Spinelli has adapted IPT for the treatment of women with antenatal depression, focusing on the role transitions and interpersonal disputes characteristic of pregnancy and motherhood. In a pilot study of 13 women (Spinelli 1997), IPT significantly reduced the severity of depressive symptoms and induced remission in all patients. Furthermore, none of the women followed after delivery ($n=10$) developed postpartum depression. Although the findings from this study are limited by its small size and lack of a control group, the results are encouraging. Not only does this modality of treatment treat the acute symptoms of depression during pregnancy; it appears to decrease risk of depression after delivery. Larger prospective studies of IPT during pregnancy are currently under way and may identify subgroups of women who are particularly responsive to such treatment.

Pharmacologic Interventions

Many reviews have been published that describe available data (from anecdotal case reports and larger prospectively derived samples) regarding risks associated with fetal exposure to antidepressants (Altshuler et al. 2001; Cohen and Rosenbaum 1997; Cohen et al. 1998; Cott and Wisner 2003). Although accumulated data over the past 30 years suggest that some antidepressants may be used safely during pregnancy (Altshuler et al. 1996; Cohen and Altshuler 1997; Wisner et al. 1999), information regarding the spectrum of attendant risks of prenatal exposure to psychotropic medications is still incomplete.

When considering the use of a psychiatric medication during pregnancy, the clinician must address four primary types of risk with respect to the developing fetus: 1) risk of pregnancy loss or miscarriage, 2) risk of organ malformation or teratogenesis, 3) risk of neonatal toxicity or withdrawal syndromes during the acute neonatal period, and 4) risk of long-term neurobehavioral sequelae (Cohen and Altshuler 1997). To provide guidance to physicians seeking information on the reproductive safety of various prescription medications, the FDA established a system that classifies medications into five risk categories (A, B, C, D, and X) based on data derived from human and animal studies. Category A medications are designated as safe for use during pregnancy, while category X drugs are contraindicated and are known to have risks to the fetus that outweigh any benefit to the patient. Most psychotropic medications are classified as category C, agents for which human studies are lacking and for which "risk cannot be ruled out." No psychotropic drugs are classified as safe for use during pregnancy (category A).

Unfortunately, this system of classification is frequently ambiguous and may sometimes be misleading. For example, certain tricyclic antidepressants (TCAs) have been labeled as category D, indicating "positive evidence of risk," although the pooled available data do not support this assertion and, in fact, suggest that these drugs are safe for use during pregnancy (Altshuler et al. 1996; Pastuszak et al. 1993). Therefore, the physician must rely on other sources of information when providing well-informed recommendations on the use of psychotropic medications during pregnancy. For obvious ethical reasons, it is not possible to conduct randomized, placebo-controlled studies on medication safety in pregnant populations. Therefore, much of the data on reproductive safety has been derived from retrospective studies and case reports, although more recent studies have used a prospective design (Chambers et al. 1996; Einarson et al. 2001a; Kulin et al. 1998; Nulman et al. 1997; Pastuszak et al. 1993).

Risk of Pregnancy Loss or Miscarriage

Recent attention has focused on whether certain antidepressants may increase the risk of early pregnancy loss. While most reports do not indicate that antidepressants increase the risk of miscarriage, several reports have suggested small increases in rates of spontaneous abortion among women treated with selective serotonin reuptake inhibitor (SSRI) and serotonin-norepinephrine reuptake inhibitor (SNRI) antidepressants during the first trimester of pregnancy (Einarson et al. 2001a; Kulin et al. 1998; Pastuszak et al. 1993). In these reports, the observed differences did not reach statistical significance; rates of miscarriage in exposed women were in the range of what would be normally expected in women with no known exposure. An alternative explanation for the finding of slightly increased risk of miscarriage in antidepressant-exposed women is that depression itself is a factor that may contribute to increasing risk of spontaneous abortion (Sugiura-Ogasawara et al. 2002). Some authors also suggest that the number of spontaneous abortions may have been overestimated, because some women taking medications at conception, when questioned during the follow-up interviews, may have chosen to report a miscarriage, when in fact they had decided to terminate their pregnancy (Einarson et al. 2001a). Further studies are needed to better define the risk of pregnancy loss.

Risk of Organ Malformation or Teratogenesis

The baseline incidence of major congenital malformations in newborns born in the United States is estimated to be 3%–4% (Fabro 1987). During the earliest stages of pregnancy, formation of major organ systems takes place and is complete within the first 12 weeks after conception. A *teratogen* is defined as an agent that interferes with this process and produces some type of organ malformation or dysfunction. Exposure to a toxic agent before 2 weeks of gestation is not associated with congenital malformations and is more likely to result in a nonviable blighted ovum (Langman 1985). For each organ or organ system, there exists a critical period during which development takes place and may be susceptible to the effects of a teratogen (Moore and Persaud 2003). For example, formation of the heart and great vessels takes place 4–9 weeks after conception. Formation of lip and palate is typically complete by week 10. Neural tube folding and closure, which form the brain and spinal cord, occur within the first 4 weeks of gestation.

To date, studies have not demonstrated a statistically increased risk of congenital malformations associated with prenatal exposure to antidepressants. Two meta-analyses combining studies with exposures to TCAs and SSRIs did not demonstrate an increase in risk of congenital malformation (Addis and Koren 2000; Altshuler et al. 1996). Data supporting the reproductive safety of fluoxetine (Chambers et al. 1996; Cohen et al. 2000; Goldstein 1995; Goldstein et al. 1991, 1997; Loebstein and Koren 1997; McElhatton et al. 1996; Nulman and Koren 1996) and citalopram (Ericson et al. 1999) are particularly robust. Four prospective studies have evaluated rates of congenital malformations in approximately 1,100 fluoxetine-exposed infants (Chambers et al. 1996; Goldstein 1995; Nulman and Koren 1996; Pastuszak et al. 1993). The postmarketing surveillance registry established by the manufacturer of fluoxetine and several other retrospective studies (McElhatton et al. 1996; Simon et al. 2002) complement these findings. These data, collected from more than 2,500 cases, indicate no increase in the risk of major congenital malformations in fluoxetine-exposed infants. Data regarding the use of citalopram come primarily from one prospective study of 969 infants with first-trimester exposure to SSRIs (including 375 exposures to citalopram) and other antidepressants (Ericson et al. 1999).

Information regarding the reproductive safety of other SSRIs, including sertraline, paroxetine, fluvoxamine, and the SNRI venlafaxine, is gradually accumulating (Ericson et al. 1999; Inman et al. 1993; Kulin et al. 1998; McElhatton et al. 1996; Simon et al. 2002). In a retrospective study of 63 infants with first-trimester exposure to paroxetine, no increase in teratogenic risk was observed (Inman et al. 1993). In another report including 150 pregnant women, the use of venlafaxine during pregnancy did not increase the rate of major malformations above the expected baseline rate. While these initial reports are reassuring, larger samples are required to establish the reproductive safety of these newer antidepressants. It has been estimated that at least 500–600 exposures to a given drug must be collected to demonstrate a twofold increase in risk for a particular malformation over what is observed in the general population (Shepard 1989). Many studies, rather than assessing outcomes in infants exposed to a single antidepressant, observed outcomes in larger samples of infants exposed to any SSRI antidepressant. In these pooled samples, no increase in the risk of malformation was observed in infants exposed to SSRIs (Ericson et al. 1999; Hendrick et al. 2003; Kulin et al. 1998; McElhatton et al. 1996; Simon et al. 2002). Although limited in terms of sample size, the data supporting the safety of SSRIs (as a class) and venlafaxine are increasingly reassuring.

Although early case reports suggested a possible association between first-trimester exposure to TCAs and limb malformation, 3 prospective and more than 10 retrospective studies have examined the risk of organ dysgenesis in over 400 cases of first-trimester exposure to TCAs (Altshuler et al. 1996; Cohen and Rosenbaum 1997; Loebstein and Koren 1997; McElhatton et al. 1996; Misri and Sivertz 1991). When evaluated on an individual basis and when pooled, these studies fail to indicate a significant association between fetal exposure to TCAs and risk of any major congenital anomaly. Among the TCAs, desipramine and nortriptyline are preferred since they are less anticholinergic and the least likely to exacerbate orthostatic hypotension that occurs during pregnancy.

While there is information to support the use of certain antidepressants, including fluoxetine, citalopram, and the TCAs, during pregnancy, there are many fewer data on the reproductive safety of other antidepressants. A recent prospective study of women taking either nefazodone ($n=89$) or trazodone ($n=58$) during the first trimester of pregnancy suggested no increase in the risk of major malformation (Einarson et al. 2003). To date, prospective data on the use of mirtazapine and duloxetine are lacking. Scant information is available regarding the reproductive safety of monoamine oxidase inhibitors (MAOIs). One study in humans described an increase in congenital malformations after prenatal exposure to tranylcypromine and phenelzine, although the sample size was extremely small (Heinonen et al. 1977). Moreover, during labor and delivery, MAOIs may produce a hypertensive crisis should tocolytic medications, such as terbutaline, be used to forestall delivery. Given this lack of data, and the cumbersome restrictions associated with their use, MAOIs are typically avoided during pregnancy.

Data regarding the use of bupropion (Wellbutrin) are incomplete and somewhat difficult to interpret. Information collected by the manufacturer (GlaxoSmithKline) includes 426 pregnancy outcomes involving first-trimester exposure to bupropion. In this sample, there were 12 outcomes that involved major malformations. This represents a 2.8% risk of congenital malformation, which is consistent with the risk observed in women with no known teratogen exposure. While this information regarding the overall risk of malformation is reassuring, the most recent report revealed that 8 of the 12 cases involved malformations of the heart and great vessels. In addition, among the 16 retrospectively reported cases of malformations in bupropion-exposed infants, 7 involved cardiac defects. While these reports may signal a potential risk, the relatively small sample size and the high percentage of cases lost to follow-up ($n=302$) make it difficult to draw conclusions regarding the impact of bupropion on the developing cardiovascular system. Further studies regarding the reproductive safety of this medication are warranted, and its use during pregnancy, while not preferable, is not absolutely contraindicated.

While no study has observed an increase in risk of *major* congenital anomaly associated with antidepressant exposure, Chambers and colleagues (1996) noted increased risk of multiple "minor" malformations in fluoxetine-exposed infants. In this study, *minor anomalies* were defined as structural defects of no cosmetic or functional importance. In addition, this report suggested that late exposure to fluoxetine was associated with premature labor and poor neonatal adaptation. Interpretation of the findings of this study is limited by several methodological difficulties (Cohen and Rosenbaum 1997). For example, the fluoxetine-exposed women and control groups differed significantly in terms of important variables such as age, presence of psychiatric illness, and exposure to other medications. In addition, nonblinded raters were utilized, and only half of the fluoxetine-exposed infants were evaluated, which raises the question of selection bias. While further data are needed to ensure clinical confidence, the data collected thus far on fluoxetine suggest that it is unlikely to be a significant human teratogen.

Risk of Neonatal Toxicity or Withdrawal Syndromes

Neonatal toxicity or *perinatal syndromes* refers to a spectrum of physical and behavioral symptoms observed in the acute neonatal period that are attributed to drug exposure at or near the time of delivery. Over the past two decades, a wide range of transient neonatal distress syndromes associated with in utero exposure to (or potentially withdrawal from) antidepressants have been described; however, given the prevalence of antidepressant use during pregnancy and the anecdotal nature of these reports, the incidence of these adverse events is, in all probability, particularly low. Anecdotal reports that attribute these syndromes to drug exposure must be interpreted cautiously, and larger samples must be studied in order to establish a causal link between exposure to a particular medication and a frank perinatal syndrome.

Various case reports have described perinatal syndromes in infants exposed to TCAs in utero. A TCA withdrawal syndrome with characteristic symptoms of jitteriness, irritability, and, less commonly, seizure (Bromiker 1994; Cowe et al. 1982; Eggermont 1973; Schimmell et al. 1991; Webster 1973) has been observed. Withdrawal seizures have been reported only with clomipramine (Bromiker 1994; Cowe et al. 1982). In addition, neonatal toxicity attributed to the anticholinergic effect of TCAs, including symptoms of functional bowel obstruction and urinary retention, has been reported (Falterman and Richardson 1980; Shearer et al. 1972). In all cases, these symptoms were transient.

The extent to which prenatal exposure to fluoxetine or other SSRIs is associated with neonatal toxicity is still unclear and has been the subject of some debate. Concerns were first raised by Chambers and colleagues (1996), who suggested that third-trimester use of fluoxetine was associated with increased risk of neonatal complications and higher rates of admission to the special care nursery. Since that time, several other studies have also described increased rates of admission to the special care nursery among SSRI-exposed infants (Casper et al. 2003; Cohen et al. 2000). More recently, several prospective studies have suggested that exposure to SSRIs at the time of delivery may be associated with other types of perinatal complications, including poor neonatal adaptation, respiratory distress, jitteriness, and feeding problems (Casper et al. 2003; Laine et al. 2003; Oberlander et al. 2004; Simon et al. 2002; Zeskind and Stephens 2004).

In addition, several reports have documented decreased gestational age and lower birth-weight in SSRI-exposed children (Chambers et al. 1996; Ericson et al. 1999; Simon et al. 2002); however, Chambers and colleagues (1996) found that only third-trimester fluoxetine exposure was associated with shorter gestational age. In general, it appears that while this effect is statistically significant, it is relatively small. For example, in the study from Simon and colleagues (2002), the mean gestational age was 38.5 weeks in the SSRI-exposed infants, compared with 39.4 weeks in the nonexposed group. Other studies do not report differences in gestational age or birth-weight in SSRI-exposed versus nonexposed children (Cohen et al. 2000; Kulin et al. 1998; Laine et al. 2003; Pastuszak et al. 1993; Suri et al. 2004; Zeskind and Stephens 2004).

One of the largest of these studies, using a large database from a group-model HMO, compared neonatal outcomes following in utero exposure to TCAs ($n=209$) or SSRIs ($n=195$) (Simon et al. 2002). There was an association between third-trimester exposure to SSRIs and lower Apgar scores; in contrast, TCA-exposed newborns did not differ from nonexposed control newborns with regard to these outcomes. Several other studies also observed lower Apgar scores in SSRI-exposed infants (Casper et al. 2003; Kallen 2004; Laine et al. 2003); however, not all studies have demonstrated differences in Apgar scores between exposed and nonexposed infants (Suri et al. 2004; Zeskind and Stephens 2004). It is reassuring to note that in the studies that demonstrated lower

Apgar scores, the difference in Apgar scores between exposed and nonexposed infants was small (less than 1 point), and the average Apgar scores in the exposed children remained high (above 7). Clinically, a score of 7 or greater at 5 minutes suggests that the baby's condition is good to excellent.

While the cumulative impression from some of these studies is that there is a small risk of neonatal distress syndrome in the setting of peripartum SSRI exposure, one of the difficulties in interpreting these data is that most of the studies do not take into consideration the impact of maternal mood on perinatal outcome. As there are reports which suggest that maternal depression may be associated with both preterm labor and poor neonatal outcomes (Orr and Miller 1995; Orr et al. 2002; Steer et al. 1992; Zuckerman et al. 1990), it is possible that depression itself (rather than the medications alone used to treat the depression) is responsible for the shorter gestation. Another significant shortcoming of the majority of these studies is that all but one (Laine et al. 2003) of the studies failed to use blind raters to assess neonatal outcomes. Most studies described observations of the child's behavior and symptoms made either by the physician or by the mother. This introduces the obvious risk of significant bias with overreporting of adverse events in children known by the rater to have had SSRI exposure.

Whether the reported symptoms of perinatal distress represent a direct effect of exposure to antidepressant or a discontinuation syndrome is not clear. In a prospective, controlled follow-up study, neonatal outcomes were assessed in 20 mothers taking 20–40 mg of either citalopram or fluoxetine and in 20 control mothers not receiving any psychotropic medication (Laine et al. 2003). The newborns were assessed by a blinded rater during the first 4 days of life and at the ages of 2 weeks and 2 months. In the exposed infants, symptoms of serotonergic overactivity were observed more frequently than in the control infants. The most frequently observed symptoms in the newborns included tremor, restlessness, and increased muscle tone. These symptoms resolved over the following 1–4 days, and no differences between the exposed and nonexposed infants at 2 weeks and 2 months were observed. Because the symptoms resolved quickly while SSRI concentrations were decreasing, the authors postulated that the symptoms were secondary to central nervous system serotonergic over-stimulation rather than to SSRI withdrawal syndrome. Several other studies have also reported transient symptoms suggestive of serotonergic overactivity, with tremulousness being one of the most commonly reported symptoms (Casper et al. 2003; Zeskind and Stephens 2004).

Other studies attribute the symptoms to antidepressant withdrawal. Case reports of neonatal withdrawal in neonates exposed to paroxetine have been published and describe transient symptoms of irritability, excessive crying, increased muscle tone, feeding problems, sleep disruption, and respiratory distress (Costei et al. 2002; Dahl et al. 1997; Nordeng et al. 2001; Stiskal et al. 2001). In a prospectively ascertained sample of 55 neonates exposed to paroxetine proximate to delivery (dose range=10–60 mg; median = 20 mg), 22% ($n=12$) had complications necessitating intensive treatment (Costei et al. 2002). The most common symptoms included respiratory distress ($n=9$), hypoglycemia ($n=2$), and jaundice ($n=1$), all of which resolved over 1–2 weeks without specific intervention. The extent to which other SSRIs (with longer half-lives) demonstrate similar risk for neonatal toxicity has yet to be explored. Furthermore, it is crucial to investigate other factors that modulate vulnerability to neonatal toxicity (e.g., prematurity, low birth-weight).

While there remains some controversy in this area, it is possible that the findings from these studies signal a potential problem. Reassuringly, the reported adverse events appear to be relatively short-lived and rarely require any type of medical intervention. Furthermore, there is no indication of longer-term problems, such as developmental delay, in children exposed to SSRIs in utero (Casper et al. 2003; Laine et al. 2003; Nulman et al. 1997, 2002; Simon et al. 2002). Clearly, further research is essential, but pending more controlled study, appropriate vigilance of exposed newborns after delivery is good clinical practice. However, it has been well documented that lowering the maintenance dosage in recurrently ill women with depression increases the risk of recurrence, which can occur on the cusp of an already high-risk period for women—namely, the postpartum period. Given the negative impact of maternal depression on the child's development, maintaining affective stability in the mother should be considered a highest and uncompromised priority. On the basis of a number of anecdotal reports of toxicity in infants born to mothers treated with antidepressants, some authors have recommended discontinuation of antidepressant medication several days or weeks prior to delivery to minimize the risk of neonatal toxicity. It is unclear at this point whether discontinuing or lowering the dosage of the mother's antidepressant shortly before delivery will reduce the risk of neonatal toxicity. Given the low incidence of neonatal toxicity with most antidepressants, this practice carries significant risk, since it withdraws treatment from patients precisely as they are about to enter the postpartum period, a time of heightened risk for developing affective illness.

In October 2004, the FDA ordered drug manufacturers to include warnings in the packaging inserts regarding the use of certain antidepressants, including the SSRIs and venlafaxine (Effexor), during pregnancy. The labels now describe a spectrum of adverse events in newborns exposed to these drugs late in the third trimester, including jitteriness, irritability, hypoglycemia, feeding difficulties, respiratory distress, abnormal muscle tone, and constant crying. Complications requiring "prolonged hospitalization, respiratory support and tube feeding" are also mentioned. While transient and relatively benign adverse events have been reported, the more serious problems, such as prolonged hospitalization and the need for respiratory support, are not well supported by any objective data in the medical literature. Listing these in the label may do little but alarm patients and physicians and fail to inform the appropriate clinical path to pursue.

The labeling changes will likely create alarm about a potential clinical syndrome that has an extremely low incidence and modest clinical significance. While it is possible that some children may experience adverse events subsequent to delivery, it is important to put these concerns within a larger context. As noted earlier, reassuringly, the reported adverse events appear to be relatively short-lived and rarely require any type of medical intervention. Furthermore, as discussed below, there is no indication of longer-term neurobehavioral problems in children exposed to

SSRIs in utero (Casper et al. 2003; Laine et al. 2003; Nulman et al. 1997, 2002; Simon et al. 2002).

Risk of Long-Term Neurobehavioral Sequelae

Because neuronal migration and differentiation occur throughout pregnancy and into the early years of life, the central nervous system remains particularly vulnerable to toxic agents throughout pregnancy. However, insults that occur after neural-tube closure and folding produce changes in behavior and function, as opposed to gross structural abnormalities. *Behavioral teratogenesis* refers to the potential of a psychotropic drug administered prenatally to cause long-term *neurobehavioral sequelae*. For example, are children who have been exposed to an antidepressant in utero at risk for cognitive or behavioral problems at a later point during development? Animal studies demonstrate changes in behavior and neurotransmitter function after prenatal exposure to a variety of psychotropic agents (Ali et al. 1986; Ansorge et al. 2004; Bonari et al. 2004; Vernadakis and Parker 1980; Vorhees et al. 1979). The extent to which these findings are of consequence to humans has yet to be demonstrated.

With regard to long-term neurobehavioral sequelae in children exposed to either fluoxetine or TCAs, the data are limited but reassuring. In a landmark study, Nulman and colleagues (1997) followed a cohort of children up to preschool age who had been exposed to either TCAs ($n=80$) or fluoxetine ($n=55$) in utero (most commonly during the first trimester), and compared these subjects to a cohort of nonexposed controls ($n=84$). Results indicated no significant differences in IQ, temperament, behavior, reactivity, mood, distractibility, or activity level between exposed and nonexposed children. In a more recent report, the same group followed a cohort of children exposed to fluoxetine ($n=40$) or TCAs ($n=47$) for the entire duration of the pregnancy and demonstrated similar results (Nulman et al. 2002). The authors concluded that their findings support the hypothesis that fluoxetine and TCAs are not behavioral teratogens. However, these data are preliminary, and clearly further investigation into the long-term neurobehavioral effects of prenatal exposure to antidepressants, as well as other psychotropic medications, is warranted.

Electroconvulsive Therapy During Pregnancy

The use of electroconvulsive therapy (ECT) during pregnancy typically raises considerable anxiety on the part of clinicians and patients. Its safety record has been well documented over the last 50 years (Goldstein et al. 1941; Impasato et al. 1964; Remick and Maurice 1978). Requests for psychiatric consultation on pregnant patients requiring ECT tend to be emergent and dramatic. For example, expeditious treatment is imperative in instances of mania or psychotic depression with suicidal thoughts and disorganized thinking during pregnancy. Such clinical situations are associated with a danger from impulsivity or self-harm. The safety and efficacy of ECT in such settings are well described, particularly when the ECT is instituted in collaboration with a multidisciplinary treatment team, including an anesthesiologist, a psychiatrist, and an obstetrician (Miller 1994; Remick and Maurice 1978; Repke and Berger 1984; Wise et al. 1984). A limited course of treatment may be sufficient followed by institution of treatment with one agent or a combination of agents, such as antidepressants, neuroleptics, benzodiazepines, or mood stabilizers.

ECT during pregnancy tends to be underused because of concerns that treatment will harm the fetus. Despite one report of placental abruption associated with the use of ECT in pregnancy (Sherer et al. 1991), considerable experience supports its safe use in severely ill gravid women. Thus, it becomes the task of the psychiatric consultant to facilitate the most clinically appropriate intervention in the face of partially informed concerns or objections.

Treatment of Anxiety Disorders During Pregnancy

The use of nonpharmacologic treatments such as CBT and supportive psychotherapy may be of great value in attenuating symptoms of anxiety in some cases (Otto et al. 1993; Robinson et al. 1992). While patients with severe illness may opt to continue to take medication during pregnancy, those with milder forms of illness may consider discontinuing treatment during pregnancy. For patients with panic disorder who wish to conceive, a slow taper of antipanic medications is recommended. Adjunctive CBT may be of some benefit in helping patients discontinue antipanic agents and may increase the time to relapse (Robinson et al. 1992). Some patients may conceive inadvertently while taking antipanic medications and may present for emergent consultation. Abrupt discontinuation of antipanic maintenance medication is not recommended, given the risk of rebound panic symptoms or a potentially serious withdrawal syndrome. However, gradual tapering of antipanic medications (i.e., >2 weeks) with adjunctive CBT may be pursued in an effort to minimize fetal exposure to medication.

For others, especially those with panic attacks associated with new-onset or recurrent panic disorder, or those with severe generalized anxiety disorder (GAD) or OCD, pharmacologic intervention may be a clinical necessity. Similarly, if a taper is unsuccessful or if symptoms recur during pregnancy, reinstitution of pharmacotherapy may be considered. Pharmacotherapy of severe anxiety during pregnancy may include treatment with benzodiazepines, TCAs, SSRIs, or SNRIs. These classes of drugs have all demonstrated efficacy in the management of GAD (Chouinard et al. 1982; Sheehan et al. 1980), panic disorder (Charney et al. 1986; Dunner et al. 1986; Gorman et al. 1987), and OCD (Goodman 1999).

For patients with severe anxiety disorder, maintenance medication may be a clinical necessity. For those with OCD, SSRIs or clomipramine is the first line of treatment. Because of the concerns regarding serious withdrawal symptoms in infants exposed to clomipramine in utero, the SSRIs are preferred. However, clomipramine may be used with close monitoring in those women who do not respond to or are unable to tolerate SSRIs. Use of the SSRIs or TCAs is a reasonable option for the management of panic disorder and GAD during pregnancy (Altshuler et al. 1996). If patients do not respond to these antidepressants, benzodiazepines may be considered (Weinstock et al. 2001).

Benzodiazepine Use in Pregnancy

Risk of Oral Cleft and Major Malformations During First-Trimester Exposure

Concerns regarding the potential association between first-trimester exposure to benzodiazepines, such as diazepam, and increased risk of oral clefts have been noted in some studies (Aarskog 1975; Safra and Oakley 1975; Saxen 1975); however, other studies do not support this association (Rosenberg et al. 1983; Shiono and Mills 1984). Early reports suggested that benzodiazepines, specifically diazepam, were associated with higher risk of cleft lip and/or cleft palate in children exposed during the first trimester. Over the next decade, investigators studied the effects of individual benzodiazepines and benzodiazepines as a class, but the studies presented considerable methodological problems: enrolled patients came from very different settings, had been exposed to different benzodiazepines at different dosages, and often had taken other psychiatric medications or illicit substances. It is therefore difficult to decide which studies are most appropriate for inclusion in a meta-analysis of benzodiazepine exposure.

One meta-analysis of benzodiazepines as a class (including diazepam, alprazolam, and clonazepam, among others) looked specifically at risk of cleft lip and/or cleft palate (Altshuler et al. 1996); there has been little concern about other malformations associated with benzodiazepines. When studies with great variability with respect to methodologic rigor were included, a small but nonetheless increased risk of oral clefts associated with first-trimester benzodiazepine exposure was noted, on the order of 0.6%—which represents a tenfold increased risk relative to the general population, where the risk of oral clefts is 6 in 10,000.

A subsequent, even larger meta-analysis examined the risk of malformations, and specifically oral clefts, across all benzodiazepines (Dolovich et al. 1998). Again, the results were mixed. In that study, the risk of oral clefts was increased, but not to the degree found in the first meta-analysis. The increase in relative risk was more modest, and differences were more discernible in the case-control than in the cohort studies. In fact, if one excluded from that meta-analysis the most profoundly flawed study (Laegreid et al. 1990), the risk estimate would be even smaller for oral cleft. Given the data regarding the risk of cleft lip and palate, some women may choose to avoid first-trimester exposure. However, benzodiazepines may be used without significant risk during the second and third trimesters, and they may offer some advantage over antidepressant treatment because they may be used as needed.

Adverse Effects During Pregnancy or Peripartum

With respect to the use of benzodiazepines during pregnancy at or about the time of labor and delivery, reports of hypotonia, neonatal apnea, neonatal withdrawal syndromes, and temperature dysregulation (Fisher et al. 1985; Gillberg 1977; Mazzi 1977; Rementaria and Blatt 1977; Rowlatt 1978; Speight 1977; Whitelaw et al. 1981) have prompted recommendations to taper and to discontinue benzodiazepines at the time of parturition. The rationale for this course is suspect for several reasons. First, given the data suggesting a risk of puerperal worsening of anxiety disorders in women with histories of panic disorder and OCD (Cohen et al. 1994b; Sichel et al. 1993a, 1993b), discontinuation of a drug at or about the time of delivery places women at risk for postpartum worsening of these disorders. Second, one report described the use of clonazepam during labor and delivery at dosages of 0.5–3.5 mg/day in a group of women with panic disorder without evidence of perinatal sequelae (Weinstock et al. 2001).

General Guidelines for Treatment of Mood and Anxiety Disorders During Pregnancy

The past decade has brought increased attention to the question of how to best manage women who suffer from psychiatric illness during pregnancy. The management of mood and anxiety disorders during pregnancy is largely guided by practical experience, with few definitive data and, for obvious ethical reasons, no controlled treatment studies to inform treatment. Clinically, the most appropriate treatment algorithm is contingent on the severity of the disorder and ultimately on the wishes of the patient. Clinicians must work collaboratively with the patient to arrive at a decision based on available information and the patient's wishes. A patient's past psychiatric history and current symptoms, as well as her attitude toward the use of psychiatric medications during pregnancy, must be carefully assessed and factored into treatment decisions.

Women with histories of mood or anxiety disorders frequently present for consultation regarding the use of psychotropic medications before pregnancy, or they may seek treatment after recurrence of illness following conception. Not infrequently, women present with the first onset of psychiatric illness during pregnancy. All decisions regarding the continuation or initiation of pharmacologic treatment during pregnancy must reflect an assessment of the following risks: 1) risk of fetal exposure to medication, 2) risk of untreated psychiatric illness in the mother, and 3) risk of relapse associated with discontinuation of maintenance treatment. The clinician should document in the medical record a discussion of each of these risks, as well as the patient's competence to understand these issues regarding treatment.

Nonpharmacologic interventions such as CBT or IPT should be considered first, as they pose the smallest risk to the fetus. When pharmacologic treatment is indicated, the clinician should attempt to select the safest medication regimen, using, if possible, medications with the largest and most complete reproductive safety profile. For both mood and anxiety disorders, SSRIs and TCAs are first-line agents; however, some women, particularly those with GAD or panic disorder, may require or prefer to use treatment with benzodiazepines. In general, medications for which there are ample data regarding reproductive safety are used preferentially. However, there may be certain situations when it is appropriate to use a medication during pregnancy even in the absence of adequate data. For example, if a woman has had a poor response to SSRIs in the past but has had a good response to a medication for which the data on reproductive safety are more limited (e.g., mirtazapine), one may consider using this less well-characterized medication during pregnancy. The decision should be made, of course, in the context of an informed conversation with the patient, with the clinician acknowledging the lack of extensive information regarding the medication's reproductive safety. Informing the decision-making process is the understanding that untreated psychiatric illness in the mother is not benign and may be associated with maternal morbidity and associated adverse effects on children. As a general principle, sustaining euthymia, even when treatment may involve use of compounds for which there are no robust data confirming safety, should be the primary goal.

With regard to optimal dosage of medication during pregnancy, the lowest effective dosage should be used. The dosage of medication needed to keep a woman well before pregnancy should be maintained across pregnancy, unless she develops symptoms of recurrent symptoms when pregnant, at which time the dose could be raised to ensure mood stability. Frequently, the clinician and patient elect to reduce the dosage of a medication during pregnancy, presumably in an effort to minimize risk to the fetus. However, this type of treatment modification may instead place the woman at greater risk for recurrent illness. During pregnancy, changes in plasma volume, as well as increases in hepatic metabolism and renal clearance, may significantly affect drug levels (Jeffries and Bochner 1988; Krauer 1985). Several investigators have described a significant reduction (up to 65%) in serum levels of TCAs during pregnancy (Altshuler et al. 1996; Wisner et al. 1993). Subtherapeutic levels were associated with depressive relapse (Altshuler et al. 1996); therefore, daily TCA dosage was increased during pregnancy to induce remission. Similarly, many women taking SSRIs during pregnancy require an increase in SSRI dosage to sustain euthymia (Hostetter et al. 2000).

In prescribing medications during pregnancy, every attempt should be made to simplify the medication regimen. For instance, the clinician may select a more sedating TCA for a woman who presents with depression and sleep disturbance, rather than using an SSRI in combination with trazodone or a benzodiazepine.

Conclusion

Mood and anxiety disorders occur commonly during pregnancy, and women with recurrent illness appear to be at high risk for relapse, particularly if maintenance treatments are decreased or discontinued. While the use of psychotropic medications during pregnancy understandably raises concerns, there are data to support the use of certain antidepressants, including fluoxetine, citalopram, and the tricyclic antidepressants. Data on the newer selective serotonin reuptake inhibitor antidepressants are gradually accumulating and are encouraging. None of the SSRIs or TCAs have been associated with an increased risk of congenital malformation. However, information on risk of either transient neonatal symptoms with attendant symptoms of jitteriness and tremulousness or long-term neurobehavioral effects remains limited.

As depression during pregnancy carries risk for both mother and child, it is crucial to recognize depression in this setting and to introduce appropriate pharmacologic *and* nonpharmacologic treatment strategies. Further data on the efficacy of nonpharmacologic and pharmacologic strategies in treating subgroups of women at variable risk are clearly needed to facilitate the most tailored treatment for these women, with interventions matched to the individual needs and wishes of patients.

References

Aarskog D: Association between maternal intake of diazepam and oral clefts (letter). Lancet 2:921, 1975

Addis A, Koren G: Safety of fluoxetine during the first trimester of pregnancy: a meta-analytical review of epidemiological studies. Psychol Med 30:89–94, 2000

Ali S, Buelkesam J, Newport L: Early neurobehavioral and neurochemical alterations in rats prenatally exposed to imipramine. Neurotoxicology 7:365–380, 1986

Altshuler LL, Cohen LS, Szuba MP, et al: Pharmacologic management of psychiatric illness in pregnancy: dilemmas and guidelines. Am J Psychiatry 153:592–606, 1996

Altshuler LL, Cohen LS, Moline ML, et al: The Expert Consensus Guideline Series. Treatment of depression in women. Postgrad Med (Spec No), March 2001, pp 1–107

Alves SE, Akbari HM, Anderson GM, et al: Neonatal ACTH administration elicits long-term changes in forebrain monoamine innervation: subsequent disruptions in hypothalamic-pituitary-adrenal and gonadal function. Ann NY Acad Sci 814:226–251, 1997

Andersson L, Sundstrom-Poromaa I, Wulff M, et al: Neonatal outcome following maternal antenatal depression and anxiety: a population-based study. Am J Epidemiol 159:872–881, 2004

Ansorge MS, Zhou M, Lira A, et al: Early-life blockade of the 5-HT transporter alters emotional behavior in adult mice. Science 306:879–881, 2004

Appleby L: Suicide during pregnancy and in the first postnatal year. BMJ 302:137–140, 1991

Beck AT, Rush AJ, Shaw BF, et al: Cognitive Therapy of Depression. New York, Guilford, 1979

Bonari L, Pinto N, Ahn E, et al: Perinatal risks of untreated depression during pregnancy. Can J Psychiatry 49:726–735, 2004

Bromiker RKL: Apparent intrauterine fetal withdrawal from clomipramine hydrochloride. JAMA 272:1722–1723, 1994

Casper RC, Fleisher BE, Lee-Ancajas JC, et al: Follow-up of children of depressed mothers exposed or not exposed to antidepressant drugs during pregnancy. J Pediatr 142:402–408, 2003

Chambers C, Johnson K, Dick L, et al: Birth outcomes in pregnant women taking fluoxetine. N Engl J Med 335:1010–1015, 1996

Charney DS, Woods SW, Goodman WK, et al: Drug treatment of panic disorder: the comparative efficacy of imipramine, alprazolam, and trazodone. J Clin Psychiatry 47:580–586, 1986

Chouinard G, Annable L, Fontaine R, et al: Alprazolam in the treatment of generalized anxiety and panic disorders: a double-blind placebo controlled study. Psychopharmacology (Berl) 77:229–233, 1982

Cohen LS, Altshuler L: Pharmacologic management of psychiatric illness during pregnancy and the postpartum period, in Psychiatric Clinics of North America Annual of Drug Therapy. Edited by Dunner D, Rosenbaum J. Philadelphia, PA, WB Saunders, 1997, pp 21–60

Cohen LS, Rosenbaum J: Birth outcomes in pregnant women taking fluoxetine (letter). N Engl J Med 336:872–873, 1997

Cohen LS, Rosenbaum JF: Psychotropic drug use during pregnancy: weighing the risks. J Clin Psychiatry 59 (suppl 2):18–28, 1998

Cohen LS, Rosenbaum JF, Heller VL: Panic attack–associated placental abruption: a case report. J Clin Psychiatry 50:266–267, 1989

Cohen LS, Sichel DA, Dimmock JA, et al: Impact of pregnancy on panic disorder: a case series. J Clin Psychiatry 55:284–288, 1994a

Cohen LS, Sichel DA, Dimmock JA, et al: Postpartum course in women with preexisting panic disorder. J Clin Psychiatry 55:289–292, 1994b

Cohen LS, Sichel DA, Faraone SV, et al: Course of panic disorder during pregnancy and the puerperium: a preliminary study. Biol Psychiatry 39:950–954, 1996

Cohen LS, Altshuler L, Heller V, et al: Psychotropic drug use in pregnancy, in The Practitioner's Guide to Psychoactive Drugs. Edited by Bassuk GA. New York, Plenum, 1998, pp 417–440

Cohen LS, Heller VL, Bailey JW, et al: Birth outcomes following prenatal exposure to fluoxetine. Biol Psychiatry 48:996–1000, 2000

Cohen LS, Nonacs RM, Bailey JW, et al: Relapse of depression during pregnancy following antidepressant discontinuation: a preliminary prospective study. Arch Women Ment Health 7:217–221, 2004a

Cohen LS, Soares C, Otto M, et al: Relapse of panic disorder during pregnancy among patients who discontinue or maintain antipanic medication: a preliminary prospective study. Presentation at the 157th annual meeting of the American Psychiatric Association, New York City, May 1–6, 2004b

Costei AM, Kozer E, Ho T, et al: Perinatal outcome following third trimester exposure to paroxetine. Arch Pediatr Adolesc Med 156:1129–1132, 2002

Cott AD, Wisner KL: Psychiatric disorders during pregnancy. Int Rev Psychiatry 15:217–230, 2003

Cowe L, Lloyd DJ, Dawling S: Neonatal convulsions caused by withdrawal from maternal clomipramine. Br Med J (Clin Res Ed) 284:1837–1838, 1982

Crandon AJ: Maternal anxiety and neonatal well-being. J Psychosom Res 23:113–115, 1979

Dahl ML, Olhager E, Ahlner J: Paroxetine withdrawal syndrome in a neonate (letter). Br J Psychiatry 171:391–392, 1997

Dayan J, Creveuil C, Herlicoviez M, et al: Role of anxiety and depression in the onset of spontaneous preterm labor. Am J Epidemiol 155:293–301, 2002

Dencker SJ, Malm U, Lepp M: Schizophrenic relapse after drug withdrawal is predictable. Acta Psychiatr Scand 73:181–185, 1986

Dolovich LR, Addis A, Vaillancourt JM, et al: Benzodiazepine use in pregnancy and major malformations or oral cleft: meta-analysis of cohort and case-control studies. BMJ 317:839–843, 1998

Dunner DL, Ishiki D, Avery DH, et al: Effect of alprazolam and diazepam on anxiety and panic attacks in panic disorder: a controlled study. J Clin Psychiatry 47:458–460, 1986

Eggermont E: Withdrawal symptoms in neonates associated with maternal imipramine therapy (letter). Lancet 2:680, 1973

Einarson A, Fatoye B, Sarkar M, et al: Pregnancy outcome following gestational exposure to venlafaxine: a multicenter prospective controlled study. Am J Psychiatry 158:1728–1730, 2001a

Einarson A, Selby P, Koren G: Abrupt discontinuation of psychotropic drugs during pregnancy: fear of teratogenic risk and impact of counselling. J Psychiatry Neurosci 26:44–48, 2001b

Einarson A, Bonari L, Voyer-Lavigne S, et al: A multicentre prospective controlled study to determine the safety of trazodone and nefazodone use during pregnancy. Can J Psychiatry 48:106–110, 2003

Ericson A, Kallen B, Wiholm B: Delivery outcome after the use of anti-depressants in early pregnancy. Eur J Clin Pharmacol 55:503–508, 1999

Evans J, Heron J, Francomb H, et al: Cohort study of depressed mood during pregnancy and after childbirth. BMJ 323:257–260, 2001

Fabro SE: Clinical Obstetrics. New York, Wiley, 1987

Falterman LG, Richardson DJ: Small left colon syndrome associated with maternal ingestion of psychotropics. J Pediatr 97:300–310, 1980

Fisher J, Edgren B, Mammel M: Neonatal apnea associated with maternal clonazepam therapy. Obstet Gynecol 66:34–35, 1985

Frautschi S, Cerulli A, Maine D: Suicide during pregnancy and its neglect as a component of maternal mortality. Int J Gynaecol Obstet 47:275–284, 1994

Gillberg C: "Floppy infant syndrome" and maternal diazepam (letter). Lancet 2:244, 1977

Gitlin M, Nuechterlein K, Subotnik KL, et al: Clinical outcome following neuroleptic discontinuation in patients with remitted recent-onset schizophrenia. Am J Psychiatry 158:1835–1842, 2001

Glover V: Maternal stress or anxiety in pregnancy and emotional development of the child. Br J Psychiatry 171:105–106, 1997

Goldstein DJ: Effects of third trimester fluoxetine exposure on the newborn. J Clin Psychopharmacol 15:417–420, 1995

Goldstein DJ, Williams ML, Pearson DK: Fluoxetine-exposed pregnancies (abstract). Clin Res 39:768A, 1991

Goldstein DJ, Sundell KL, Corbin LA: Birth outcomes in pregnant women taking fluoxetine. N Engl J Med 336:872–873, 1997

Goldstein H, Weinberg J, Sankstone M: Shock therapy in psychosis complicating pregnancy, a case report. Am J Psychiatry 98:201–202, 1941

Goodman WK: Obsessive-compulsive disorder: diagnosis and treatment. J Clin Psychiatry 18:27–32, 1999

Gorman JM, Liebowitz MR, Fyer AJ, et al: An open trial of fluoxetine in the treatment of panic attacks. J Clin Psychopharmacol 7:329–332, 1987

Gotlib IH, Whiffen VE, Mount JH, et al: Prevalence rates and demographic characteristics associated with depression in pregnancy and the postpartum period. J Consult Clin Psychol 57:269–274, 1989

Heinonen O, Sloan D, Shapiro S: Birth Defects and Drugs in Pregnancy. Littleton, MA, PSG Publishing, 1977

Hendrick V, Smith LM, Suri R, et al: Birth outcomes after prenatal exposure to antidepressant medication. Am J Obstet Gynecol 188:812–815, 2003

Heron J, O'Connor TG, Evans J, et al: The course of anxiety and depression through pregnancy and the postpartum in a community sample. J Affect Disord 80:65–73, 2004

Hostetter A, Stowe ZN, Strader JR Jr, et al: Dose of selective serotonin uptake inhibitors across pregnancy: clinical implications. Depress Anxiety 11:51–57, 2000

Impasato DJ, Gabriel AR, Lardara M: Electric and insulin shock therapy during pregnancy. Dis Nerv Syst 25:542–546, 1964

Inman W, Kobotu K, Pearce G, et al: Prescription event monitoring of paroxetine. PEM Reports PXL 1206:1–44, 1993

Istvan J: Stress, anxiety, and birth outcome: a critical review of the evidence. Psychol Bull 100:331–348, 1986

Jeffries WS, Bochner F: The effect of pregnancy on drug pharmacokinetics. Med J Aust 149:675–677, 1988

Kallen B: Neonate characteristics after maternal use of antidepressants in late pregnancy. Arch Pediatr Adolesc Med 158:312–316, 2004

Keller MB, Lavori PW, Lewis C, et al: Predictors of relapse in major depressive disorder. JAMA 250:3299–3309, 1983

Keller MB, Klerman GL, Lavori PW, et al: Long-term outcome of episodes of major depression: clinical and public health significance. JAMA 252:788–792, 1984

Kessler RC, McGonagle KA, Swartz M, et al: Sex and depression in the National Comorbidity Survey, I: lifetime prevalence, chronicity and recurrence. J Affect Disord 29:85–96, 1993

Klein M, Essex M: Pregnant or depressed? The effects of overlap between symptoms of depression and somatic complaints of pregnancy on rates of major depression in the second trimester. Depression 2:308–314, 1995

Klerman GL, Weissman MM, Rounsaville BJ, et al: Interpersonal Psychotherapy of Depression. New York, Basic Books, 1984

Krauer B: Pharmacotherapy during pregnancy: emphasis on pharmacokinetics, in Drug Therapy During Pregnancy (Butterworth's International Medical Reviews: Obstetrics and Gynecology, Vol 2). Edited by Eskes T, Finster M. London, Butterworth-Heinemann, 1985, pp 9–31

Kulin N, Pastuszak A, Sage S, et al: Pregnancy outcome following maternal use of the new selective serotonin reuptake inhibitors: a prospective controlled multicenter study. JAMA 279:609–610, 1998

Kupfer D, Frank E, Perel J, et al: Five-year outcome for maintenance therapies in recurrent depression. Arch Gen Psychiatry 49:769–773, 1992

Laegreid L, Olegard R, Conradi N, et al: Congenital malformations and maternal consumption of benzodiazepines: a case-control study. Dev Med Child Neurol 32:432–441, 1990

Laine K, Heikkinen T, Ekblad U, et al: Effects of exposure to selective serotonin reuptake inhibitors during pregnancy on serotonergic symptoms in newborns and cord blood monoamine and prolactin concentrations. Arch Gen Psychiatry 60:720–726, 2003

Langman J: Human development: normal and abnormals, in Medical Embryology, 5th Edition. Edited by Langman J. Baltimore, MD, Williams & Wilkins, 1985, p 123

Loebstein R, Koren G: Pregnancy outcome and neurodevelopment of children exposed in utero to psychoactive drugs: the Motherisk experience. J Psychiatry Neurosci 22:192–196, 1997

Marcus SM, Flynn HA, Blow FC, et al: Depressive symptoms among pregnant women screened in obstetrics settings. J Womens Health (Larchmt) 12:373–380, 2003

Marzuk M, Tardiff K, Leon AC, et al: Lower risk of suicide during pregnancy. Am J Psychiatry 154:122–123, 1997

Mazzi E: Possible neonatal diazepam withdrawal: a case report. Am J Obstet Gynecol 129:586–587, 1977

McElhatton P, Garbis H, Elefant E, et al: The outcome of pregnancy in 689 women exposed to therapeutic doses of antidepressants: a collaborative study of the European Network of Teratology Information Services (ENTIS). Reprod Toxicol 10:285–294, 1996

Miller LJ: Use of electroconvulsive therapy during pregnancy. Hosp Community Psychiatry 45:444–450, 1994

Misri S, Sivertz K: Tricyclic drugs in pregnancy and lactation: a preliminary report. Int J Psychiatry Med 21:157–171, 1991

Moore KL, Persaud TVN: The Developing Human: Clinically Oriented Embryology, 7th Edition. Philadelphia, PA, WB Saunders, 2003

Mueller TI, Leon AC, Keller MB, et al: Recurrence after recovery from major depressive disorder during 15 years of observational follow-up. Am J Psychiatry 156:1000–1006, 1999

Murray L: The impact of postnatal depression on infant development. J Child Psychol Psychiatry 33:543–561, 1992

Murray L: Postpartum depression and child development. Psychol Med 27:253–260, 1997

Nordeng H, Lindemann R, Perminov KV: Neonatal withdrawal syndrome after in utero exposure to selective serotonin reuptake inhibitors. Acta Paediatr 90:288–291, 2001

Northcott CJ, Stein MB: Panic disorder in pregnancy. J Clin Psychiatry 55:539–542, 1994

Nulman I, Koren G: The safety of fluoxetine during pregnancy and lactation. Teratology 53:304–308, 1996

Nulman I, Rovet J, Stewart D, et al: Neurodevelopment of children exposed in utero to antidepressant drugs. N Engl J Med 336:258–262, 1997

Nulman I, Rovet J, Stewart DE, et al: Child development following exposure to tricyclic antidepressants or fluoxetine throughout fetal life: a prospective, controlled study. Am J Psychiatry 159:1889–1895, 2002

Oberlander TF, Misri S, Fitzgerald RN, et al: Pharmacologic factors associated with transient neonatal symptoms following prenatal psychotropic medication exposure. J Clin Psychiatry 65:230–237, 2004

O'Connor TG, Heron J, Golding J, et al: Maternal antenatal anxiety and behavioural/emotional problems in children: a test of a programming hypothesis. J Child Psychol Psychiatry 44:1025–1036, 2003

O'Hara MW: Social support, life events, and depression during pregnancy and the pueperium. Arch Gen Psychiatry 43:569–573, 1986

O'Hara MW: Postpartum Depression: Causes and Consequences. New York, Springer, 1995

O'Hara MW, Neunaber DJ, Zekoski EM: A prospective study of postpartum depression: prevalence, course, and predictive factors. J Abnorm Psychol 93:158–171, 1984

O'Hara MW, Zekoski EM, Philipps LH, et al: Controlled prospective study of postpartum mood disorders: comparison of childbearing and nonchildbearing women. J Abnorm Psychol 99:3–15, 1990

O'Hara MW, Schlechte JA, Lewis DA, et al: Controlled prospective study of postpartum mood disorders: psychological, environmental, and hormonal factors. J Abnorm Psychol 100:63–73, 1991

Orr S, Miller C: Maternal depressive symptoms and the risk of poor pregnancy outcome: review of the literature and preliminary findings. Epidemiol Rev 17:165–171, 1995

Orr S, James SA, Blackmore Prince C: Maternal prenatal depressive symptoms and spontaneous preterm births among African-American women in Baltimore, Maryland. Am J Epidemiol 156:797–802, 2002

Otto M, Pollack M, Sachs G, et al: Discontinuation of benzodiazepine treatment: efficacy of cognitive-behavioral therapy for patients with panic disorder. Am J Psychiatry 150:1485–1490, 1993

Pastuszak A, Schick-Boschetto B, Zuber C, et al: Pregnancy outcome following first-trimester exposure to fluoxetine (Prozac). JAMA 269: 2246–2248, 1993

Post R: Transduction of psychosocial stress into the neurobiology of recurrent affective disorder. Am J Psychiatry 149:999–1010, 1992

Rementaria JL, Blatt K: Withdrawal symptoms in neonates from intrauterine exposure to diazepam. J Pediatr 90:123–126, 1977

Remick RA, Maurice WL: ECT in pregnancy (letter). Am J Psychiatry 135:761–762, 1978

Repke JT, Berger NG: Electroconvulsive therapy in pregnancy. Obstet Gynecol 63(suppl):39S–40S, 1984

Robinson L, Walker JR, Anderson D: Cognitive-behavioural treatment of panic disorder during pregnancy and lactation. Can J Psychiatry 37:623–626, 1992

Rosenberg L, Mitchell AA, Parsells JL, et al: Lack of relation of oral clefts to diazepam use during pregnancy. N Engl J Med 309:1282–1285, 1983

Rowlatt R: Effect of maternal diazepam on the newborn. BMJ 1:985, 1978

Roy-Byrne PP, Dager SR, Cowley DS, et al: Relapse and rebound following discontinuation of benzodiazepine treatment of panic attacks: alprazolam versus diazepam. Am J Psychiatry 146:860–865, 1989

Safra MJ, Oakley GP: Association between cleft lip with or without cleft palate and prenatal exposure to diazepam. Lancet 2:478–480, 1975

Saxen I: Association between oral clefts and drugs taken during pregnancy. Int J Epidemiol 4:37–44, 1975

Schimmell MS, Katz EZ, Shaag Y, et al: Toxic neonatal effects following maternal clomipramine therapy. J Toxicol Clin Toxicol 29:479–484, 1991

Shearer WT, Schreiner RL, Marshall RE: Urinary retention in a neonate secondary to maternal ingestion of nortriptyline. J Pediatr 81:570–572, 1972

Sheehan DV, Ballenger J, Jacobsen G: Treatment of endogenous anxiety with phobic, hysterical and hypochondriacal symptoms. Arch Gen Psychiatry 37:51–59, 1980

Shepard T: Catalog of Teratogenic Agents. Baltimore, MD, Johns Hopkins University Press, 1989

Sherer DM, D'Amico LD, Warshal DP, et al: Recurrent mild abruptio placentae occurring immediately after repeated electroconvulsive therapy in pregnancy. Am J Obstet Gynecol 165:652–653, 1991

Shiono PH, Mills IL: Oral clefts and diazepam use during pregnancy (letter). N Engl J Med 311:919–920, 1984

Sichel DA, Cohen LS, Dimmock JA, et al: Postpartum obsessive compulsive disorder: a case series. J Clin Psychiatry 54:156–159, 1993a

Sichel DA, Cohen LS, Rosenbaum JF, et al: Postpartum onset of obsessive-compulsive disorder. Psychosomatics 34:277–279, 1993b

Simon G, Cunningham M, Davis R: Outcomes of prenatal antidepressant exposure. Am J Psychiatry 159:2055–2061, 2002

Speight A: Floppy infant syndrome and maternal diazepam and/or nitrazepam (letter). Lancet 2:878, 1977

Spinelli M: Interpersonal psychotherapy for depressed antepartum women: a pilot study. Am J Psychiatry 154:1028–1030, 1997

Steer RA, Scholl TO, Hediger ML, et al: Self-reported depression and negative pregnancy outcomes. J Clin Epidemiol 45:1093–1099, 1992

Stiskal JA, Kulin N, Koren G, et al: Neonatal paroxetine withdrawal syndrome. Arch Dis Child Fetal Neonatal Ed 84:F134–F135, 2001

Sugiura-Ogasawara M, Furukawa TA, Nakano Y, et al: Depression as a potential causal factor in subsequent miscarriage in recurrent spontaneous aborters. Hum Reprod 17:2580–2584, 2002

Suppes T, Baldessarini RJ, Faedda GL, et al: Risk of recurrence following discontinuation of lithium treatment in bipolar disorder. Arch Gen Psychiatry 48:1082–1088, 1991

Suri R, Altshuler L, Hendrick V, et al: The impact of depression and fluoxetine treatment on obstetrical outcome. Arch Women Ment Health 7:193–200, 2004

Teixeira JM, Fisk NM, Glover V: Association between maternal anxiety in pregnancy and increased uterine artery resistance index: cohort based study. BMJ 318:153–157, 1999

Vernadakis A, Parker KK: Drugs and the developing central nervous system. Pharmacol Ther 11:593–647, 1980

Viguera AC, Baldessarini RJ, Hegarty JD, et al: Clinical risk following abrupt and gradual withdrawal of maintenance neuroleptic treatment. Arch Gen Psychiatry 54:49–55, 1997

Viguera AC, Baldessarini RJ, Friedberg J: Discontinuing antidepressant treatment in major depression. Harv Rev Psychiatry 5:293–306, 1998

Vorhees C, Brunner R, Butcher R: Psychotropic drugs as behavioral teratogens. Science 205:1220–1225, 1979

Webster PAC: Withdrawal symptoms in neonates associated with maternal antidepressant therapy. Lancet 2:318–319, 1973

Weinberg M, Tronick E: The impact of maternal psychiatric illness on infant development. J Clin Psychiatry 59 (suppl 2):53–61, 1998

Weinstock L, Cohen LS, Bailey JW, et al: Obstetrical and neonatal outcome following clonazepam use during pregnancy: a case series. Psychother Psychosom 3:158–162, 2001

Whitelaw AG, Cummings AJ, McFadyen IR: Effect of maternal lorazepam on the neonate. Br Med J (Clin Res Ed) 282:1106–1108, 1981

Wise MG, Ward SC, Townsend-Parchman W, et al: Case report of ECT during high-risk pregnancy. Am J Psychiatry 141:99–101, 1984

Wisner KL, Perel JM, Wheeler SB: Tricyclic dose requirements across pregnancy. Am J Psychiatry 150:1541–1542, 1993

Wisner KL, Gelenberg AJ, Leonard H, et al: Pharmacologic treatment of depression during pregnancy. JAMA 282:1264–1269, 1999

Zeskind P, Stephens L: Maternal selective serotonin reuptake inhibitor use during pregnancy and newborn neurobehavior. Pediatrics 113: 368–375, 2004

Zuckerman BS, Amaro H, Bauchner H, et al: Depression during pregnancy: relationship to prior health behaviors. Am J Obstet Gynecol 160:1107–1111, 1989

Zuckerman BS, Bauchner H, Parker S, et al: Maternal depressive symptoms during pregnancy, and newborn irritability. J Dev Behav Pediatr 11:190–194, 1990

Chapter 3

Management of Bipolar Disorder During Pregnancy and the Postpartum Period

Weighing the Risks and Benefits

Adele C. Viguera, M.D.
Lee S. Cohen, M.D.
Ruta M. Nonacs, M.D., Ph.D.
Ross J. Baldessarini, M.D.

Bipolar disorder (BD) is a serious psychiatric illness that occurs in 0.5%–1.5% of individuals in the United States (Kessler et al. 1994). For women, illness onset tends to occur during the reproductive years. For those affected, the disorder is a significant source of distress, disability, loss of life through suicide, and burden on relatives and other caregivers. Substantial evidence indicates that BD is a chronic condition characterized by high rates of relapse, suicide, persistent subsyndromal morbidity, and significant psychosocial dysfunction (Coryell et al. 1993; Dion et al. 1988; Gitlin et al. 1995; Goodwin and Jamison 1990; Strakowski et al. 2000). Prevention and treatment of this illness is particularly germane to women of reproductive age. Despite the undoubtedly great clinical importance of the female reproductive life cycle (the menstrual cycle, pregnancy, postpartum, breast-feeding, and menopause), remarkably little is known about its impact on the course and treatment of BD.

Typically, women with BD encounter significant obstacles from the professional community with respect to pregnancy; they are often counseled to avoid pregnancy or to terminate an established pregnancy to avoid either exposure to potentially teratogenic medications or risk of recurrent illness (Cohen et al. 1994). Women with BD seeking prepregnancy consultation regarding management of their mood disorder during pregnancy were surveyed at a tertiary-care hospital. Of the sample, 45% reported having been advised to avoid pregnancy altogether by a psychiatrist or another mental health professional (Viguera et al. 2002a). Following prepregnancy consultation, however, 63% reported they decided to pursue pregnancy, and 37% decided to avoid pregnancy. The most commonly cited reasons for deciding not to pursue pregnancy were fears that medication would adversely affect fetal development and that illness would recur if maintenance medication was discontinued.

Physicians caring for women with BD who are either contemplating or experiencing pregnancy face a clinical challenge: to minimize risk to the fetus while limiting the morbidity in the mother and her offspring that might result from untreated psychiatric illness. Patients and their clinicians must face the difficult reality that decisions either to use or to not use medication are both potentially associated with complications. Decisions about what constitutes reasonable risk during pregnancy require shared responsibility but ultimately rest with the informed patient. Such informed choices, coupled with close psychiatric follow-up and coordinated care with the obstetrician, are components of a model to optimize the clinical care of patients with BD during pregnancy.

In the chapter, we review the available information on the course of BD in pregnancy, as well as the reproductive safety data of the major mood stabilizers. We also present guidelines for the management of BD in pregnancy and the postpartum period.

Risk and Course of Bipolar Disorder During Pregnancy

There is wide agreement that the early postpartum is a period of unusually high risk of illness recurrence in patients with BD and other psychiatric illness (Kendell et al. 1987; Lier et al. 1989). In his classic early descriptions of the manic-depressive syndrome, Kraepelin (1921) observed that attacks of mania and melancholia were common in pregnancy but were even more common following childbirth. This general impression was sustained over the past century. In contrast, risks associated with pregnancy remain less well characterized, and there is conflicting evidence as to whether pregnancy alters the risk of recurrence of major affective illness in women. Some clinical observations suggest that pregnancy may reduce the risk of acute psychiatric illness and specifically protect against recurrences of BD and psychotic disorder (McNeil et al. 1984; Sharma and Persad 1995; Targum et al. 1979). Other studies have found that rates of hospitalization are either somewhat lower during pregnancy than at other times or unchanged (Kendell et al. 1987, Lier et al. 1989; Nott 1982; Pugh et al. 1963; Terp 1998), but these studies did not examine morbidity in nonhospitalized pregnant women with BD specifically.

Grof and colleagues (2000) presented findings suggestive of an apparent protective effect of pregnancy on the course of lithium-responsive type I BD. They described a benign course, and even improvement, during pregnancy, basing their results on comparisons made before and after pregnancy in women whose illness could be managed for prolonged periods without mood-stabilizing medication. Although these findings were proposed to support the view that pregnancy may prevent recurrences of BD, the sample may not have been representative of broader groups of women with BD (Viguera et al. 2002b). Moreover, other recent research and growing clinical experience suggest that pregnancy probably does not consistently protect against recurrences of mania or major depression in women with BD; rather, it is often a time of substantial risk of relapse, particularly following discontinuation of ongoing mood-stabilizing maintenance treatment (Blehar et al. 1998; Finnerty et al. 1996; Viguera et al. 2000). Notably, in a large, well-characterized clinical sample of women with BD, Blehar and colleagues (1998) found that nearly one-half had experienced episodes of major affective illness during at least one pregnancy. More recently, Freeman and colleagues (2002) also found that approximately one-half of a sample of women with BD became symptomatic during pregnancy.

We recently analyzed the course of types I and II BD in an international sample of 101 age-matched, pregnant ($n=42$) and nonpregnant ($n=59$) women who discontinued lithium maintenance treatment. Of this sample, 52% of the pregnant women and 58% of the nonpregnant women experienced a recurrence of BD, with indistinguishable time courses, based on survival analysis for 40 weeks (Viguera et al. 2000). In contrast, only 21% of the entire sample had had a recurrence within the preceding year of treatment. Risks were similar with types I and II BD but significantly higher following four or more prior episodes and after abrupt or rapid (<2 weeks) discontinuation of lithium. These findings are consistent with the view that pregnancy may have little effect on recurrence risk in patients with BD or that discontinuing maintenance treatment itself represents a major, perhaps dominant, stressor. That discontinuing lithium maintenance treatment, or even sharply decreasing the dosage (especially if done abruptly), has a deleterious impact is strongly supported by a series of studies (Baldessarini et al. 1996, 1997, 1999; Faedda et al. 1993; Lapierre et al. 1980; Rosenbaum et al. 1994; Suppes et al. 1991, 1993; Viguera et al. 2000) but remains unstudied with respect to alternative mood-stabilizing treatments.

These studies seem to suggest that any protective effects of pregnancy on risk of recurrences of mania or depression in women with BD are limited and probably insufficient to protect most patients from recurrence risks that follow discontinuation of ongoing maintenance mood-stabilizing treatment. To some extent, risk may be predicted by the past history of illness frequency or severity and, similarly, by a history of prolonged wellness or proven ability to tolerate long periods without mood-stabilizing treatment. Clearly, more studies that control specifically for past illness, DSM diagnostic subtypes (i.e., type I, type II, and rapid-cycling), and treatment status are required to clarify the course of BD during pregnancy.

Risk and Course of Bipolar Disorder During the Postpartum Period

In contrast to the course of BD during pregnancy, for which the data are sparse, the course of this disorder in the postpartum period has received more systematic study. This period has been recognized consistently for more than a century as a time of heightened vulnerability to relapse of mood disorders, although quantitative specification of that risk remains inconsistent. Among women with BD, recurrence rates in the postpartum (i.e., 3–6 months after delivery) have ranged from 20% to 80% (Blehar 1995; Bratfos and Haug 1966; Brockington et al. 1981; Davidson and Robertson 1985; Freeman et al. 2002; Kendell et al. 1987; Klompenhouwer and van Hulst 1991; Kraepelin 1921; Reich and Winokur 1970; Rhode and Marneros 2000; Viguera et al. 2000). Of interest, these rates have tended, in more recent studies, to increase to well above 50% (with rates ranging from 67% to 82%), perhaps reflecting more reliable diagnosis and greater interest in the problems (see Blehar 1995; Freeman et al. 2002; Rhode and Marneros 2000; Viguera et al. 2000).

BD is also closely associated with postpartum psychosis (Brockington et al. 1982; Platz and Kendell 1988; Stewart et al. 1991). Several studies have demonstrated that women presenting with postpartum psychosis often go on to develop a BD (see Rhode and Marneros 2000). Postpartum psychosis is a rare condition in the general population, with incidence estimated at 1–2 per 1,000 (0.1%–0.2%). However, for women with BD, the risk may be increased to 100–200 per 1,000 (10%–20%) (Brockington et al. 1982; Platz and Kendell 1988; Stewart et al. 1991). Postpartum psychosis is characterized by rapid onset of symptoms, often within the first 48–72 hours after delivery. Patients with postpartum psychosis may present with a delirium-like condition that is often indistinguishable from manic psychosis. Postpartum psychosis is a psychiatric emergency associated with high rates of infanticide and suicide (D'Orban 1979); it requires expeditious, aggressive treatment with a mood stabilizer and neuroleptic agents or electroconvulsive therapy. Among women with a previous history of postpartum psychosis who have a subsequent pregnancy, risk of a recurrent episode of postpartum psychosis is estimated to be as high as 90% (Austin 1992; Stewart 1988; Stewart et al. 1991).

Several investigators have evaluated the extent to which treatment can attenuate this high postpartum recurrence risk (Cohen et al. 1995; Stewart et al. 1991). Most of this research concerns use of lithium prophylaxis. When lithium was given either several weeks prior to delivery or immediately postpartum, the risk of postpartum recurrence of BD was reduced on average by three- to fivefold, compared with the risk in untreated women (Abou-Saleh and Coppen 1983; Austin 1992; Cohen et al. 1995; Stewart 1988; Stewart et al. 1991; Targum et al. 1979; van Gent and Verhoeven 1992). These reports concerning lithium leave open important questions about optimal dosages and treatment timing, and direct comparisons with the effectiveness of alternative treatments have not been reported. A preliminary study of 11 women with BD found that introducing divalproex even shortly after delivery resulted in fewer recurrences than were reported in untreated but otherwise similar women (Wisner 1998). In view of the very limited research on this important problem, further systematic study of perinatal and postpartum prophylaxis with anticonvulsants, atypical antipsychotic drugs, and nonpharmacologic interventions is urgently needed.

Potential Risks of Pharmacotherapy During Pregnancy

Clinicians face particularly urgent challenges when a woman with BD plans to conceive or becomes pregnant. Although data accumulated over the last 30 years suggest that some medications may be used safely during pregnancy (Altshuler et al. 1996; Cohen and Altshuler 1997), our knowledge regarding the risks of prenatal exposure to psychotropic medications is incomplete. All psychotropics diffuse readily across the placenta, and no psychotropic drug has been approved by the U.S. Food and Drug Administration (FDA) for use during pregnancy. To guide physicians seeking information on the reproductive safety of various prescription medications, the FDA established a system that classifies medications into five risk categories (A, B, C, D, and X) based on data derived from human and animal studies. Category A medications are designated as safe for use during pregnancy, whereas category X drugs are contraindicated and are known to have risks to the fetus that outweigh any benefit to the patient. Most psychotropic medications are classified as category C: agents for which human studies are lacking and "risk cannot be ruled out." No psychotropic drugs are classfied as category A (safe for use during pregnancy).

This classification system is frequently ambiguous and sometimes may be misleading. Therefore, physicians must rely on other sources of information when providing recommendations on the use of psychotropic medications during pregnancy (Altshuler et al. 1996; Briggs et al. 1998; Cohen et al. 1994). For obvious ethical reasons, it is not possible to conduct randomized, placebo-controlled studies on medication safety in pregnant populations. Accordingly, most of the available information about reproductive safety of drugs derives from case reports and retrospective studies, with very few reports involving prospective designs (Chambers et al. 1996; Nulman et al. 1997; Pastuszak et al. 1993).

It is important to emphasize that random fetal anomalies are remarkably common and represent a high background rate against which any teratogenic effects specific to psychotropic agents are to be compared. The baseline incidence of major congenital malformations in newborns born in the United States is estimated to be between 3% and 4% of live births (Fabro 1987). Basic formation of major organ systems takes place early in pregnancy and is virtually complete within the first 12 weeks after conception. It is important to point out that pregnancy often is not confirmed until more than 6–8 weeks into the first trimester—a critical time of major organ development.

Teratogens are agents, including drugs, that interfere with the normal process of organ development to produce malformations of varying severity. Each organ system appears to be vulnerable to teratogenic effects during relatively specific and well-defined periods of time (Moore and Persaud 1998). It is important to note that there is a 2-week difference between embryonic dating and gestational dating, which is the current convention of dating based on date of last menstrual period. *Embryonic age* is based on the date of conception. Since this date can be difficult to determine, gestational dating is preferred. For example, formation of the heart and great vessels takes place from 5–10 weeks after the last menstrual period. Formation of the lip and palate is typically complete by weeks 8–14. Neural-tube folding and closure, which form the brain and spinal cord, occur within the first 5–7 weeks of gestation. Exposure to a toxic agent before 2 weeks of gestation is not associated with congenital malformations and is more likely to result in a nonviable blighted ovum (Sadler 1985).

Fetal Risks Associated With Mood-Stabilizing Agents

Lithium

Since the early 1970s, there has been concern regarding the association between prenatal exposure to lithium and risk of major congenital anomalies. Reports from an early database, the International Register of Lithium Babies, derived from a voluntary physician-reporting system described increased rates of cardiovascular malformations (most notably, Ebstein's anomaly) in lithium-exposed infants (Nora et al. 1974; Schou et al. 1973; Weinstein and Goldfield 1975). Ebstein's anomaly is characterized by right ventricular hypoplasia and downward displacemnt of the tricuspid valve. The risk for this malformation in infants with first-trimester lithium exposure was initially determined to be 400 times higher than the spontaneous rate of about 1 in 20,000 live births found in the general population (Nora et al. 1974; Schou et al. 1973; Weinstein and Goldfield 1975). However, the reliability of these estimates is highly suspect in view of the almost-certain selective reporting of adverse outcomes to such registers. Nonetheless, the ratio of cardiovascular malformations to all anomalies was high, and this left the suspicion that a potentially significant problem existed (Weinstein and Goldfield 1975).

More recent controlled epidemiologic studies suggest a real, but more modest, teratogenic risk of Ebstein's anomalies associated with first-trimester lithium exposure (Edmonds and Oakley 1990; Jacobson et al. 1992; Kallen and Tandberg 1983; Zalstein et al. 1990). From a pooled analysis of the data, Cohen and others estimated the risk of Ebstein's anomaly following first-trimester exposure to be between 1 in 2,000 (0.05%) and 1 in 1,000 (0.1%) (Cohen et al. 1994). Reported rates of other cogenital cardiovascular defects among lithium-exposed infants, based on relatively well-designed studies, have been in the range of 0.9% to 12% (Cohen et al. 1994; Jacobson et al. 1992; Kallen and Tandberg 1983). Although the estimated risk of Ebstein's anomaly in lithium-exposed infants is 10–20 times higher than that observed in the general population (1 in 20,000), the absolute risk is small, and lithium remains the safest mood stabilizer for use during pregnancy. Prenatal screening with high-resolution ultrasound and fetal echocardiography is recommended at around week 16–18 of gestation to screen for cardiac anomalies (Cohen et al. 1994; Yonkers 1998).

Additional risks of lithium use later in pregnancy include reported neonatal toxicity in offspring exposed to lithium during labor and delivery. These reports include several cases of muscular hypotonia with impaired breathing and cyanosis, often referred to as "floppy baby" syndrome (see Ananth 1976; Schou and Amdisen 1975; Woody et al. 1971; Yonkers 1998). Isolated cases of neonatal hypothyroidism and nephrogenic diabetes insipidus have also been described (Ananth 1976; Yonkers 1998). A naturalistic survey of women who were treated with lithium found no direct evidence of neonatal toxicity in newborns whose mothers had received lithium either during pregnancy or during labor and delivery (Cohen et al. 1995). A limited amount of data are available regarding behavioral outcomes of children exposed to lithium in utero. A 5-year follow-up investigation of children exposed to lithium during the second and third trimesters of pregnancy ($n=60$) found no significant behavioral problems (Schou 1976).

Anticonvulsants

Compared with lithium, anticonvulsants may pose a more serious teratogenic risk. While most of the data on the reproductive safety of anticonvulsants derive from patients with epilepsy rather than BD, more recent data suggest that it is the exposure to the anticonvulsant medication per se, as opposed to the underlying seizure disorder, that contributes to the higher rate of congenital malformation (Holmes et al. 2001). Fetal exposure to anticonvulsants is associated not only with multiple congenital anomalies but also with relatively high rates of serious central nervous system (CNS) lesions, including irreparable and often crippling spina bifida. Exposure to carbamazepine in utero is associated with a 0.5%–1% risk for neural tube defects (Rosa 1991). Infants exposed to carbamazepine prenatally are also at increased risk for developing craniofacial abnormalities, microcephaly, and growth retardation (Holmes 1990; Rosa 1991). It is not known whether the new derivative, oxcarbazepine, is associated with similar fetal risks (Devinsky 2000).

Among anticonvulsants used to treat BD, valproic acid and its various derivatives and preparations, including divalproex, may be even more serious teratogens, with rates of neural tube defects in the range of 1% to 5%—about 50 times above the base rates of about .05% in the general population (Northrup and Volcik 2000; Omtzigt et al. 1992; Robert and Guibaud 1982). These risks are of particular concern because formation of the neural tube occurs within the first month of gestation, often before the diagnosis of pregnancy has been made. Moreover, limiting the risk of neural tube defects by administering supplemental folate requires at least a month of treatment before pregnancy. Whether supplemental folate can attentuate the risk of neural tube defects in the setting of anticonvulsant exposure has not been examined. Despite the dearth of data, however, supplemental folic acid (4 mg daily) is recommended.

Prenatal exposure to valproic acid has also been associated with characteristic craniofacial abnormalities, cardiovascular malformations, limb defects, and genital anomalies, as well as other CNS structural abnormalities, including hydrocephalus (Clayton-Smith and Donnai 1995; Lammer et al. 1987; Lindhout and Meinardi 1984; Omtzigt et al. 1992; Robert and Guibaud 1982). Specific risk factors for teratogenesis include high maternal daily dosage or serum concentrations of anticonvulsant, low folate levels, and exposure to multiple anticonvulsants (Lindhout and Omtzigt 1994; Nakane et al. 1980; Omtzigt et al. 1992).

Information regarding possible neurobehavioral sequelae of anticonvulsant exposure is very limited. There is no evidence to suggest an increased risk of mental retardation, but there have been suggestions that antenatal exposure to anticonvulsants may produce subtle cognitive effects even with second- and third-trimester exposure (Reinisch et al. 1995; Scolnik et al. 1994). Data also suggest that cognitive changes may occur even with late third-trimester exposure (Reinisch et al. 1995). In one study, prenatal exposure to carbamazepine did not appear to be associated with neurobehavioral dysfunction (Scolnik et al. 1994). In another study, however, there were clear cognitive deficits (i.e., depressed IQ scores and developmental delay) noted in children exposed to carbamazepine compared with nonexposed children (Holmes 1990; Jones et al. 1989).

The information on the reproductive safety of newer anticonvulsants used to treat BD, including lamotrigine, gabapentin, oxcarbazepine, and topiramate, is still very limited. Available data are limited to a few case reports pertaining to such drugs, given alone or generally in combination with other anticonvulsants, and again, almost always to women with epilepsy. The estimated risk of malformations with lamotrigine monotherapy during the first trimester, based on data from the Lamotrigine Pregnancy Registry (2001), established by the manufacturer, was 2.5%, and data from the United Kingdom Independent Prospective Pregnancy Registry suggest a similar risk with monotherapy exposure (Murrow et al. 2001). While there appears to be no consistent pattern of birth defects in these registries, the number of pregnancies accumulated to date represents a sample of insufficient size for reaching definitive conclusions regarding teratogenic risks of lamotrigine. In an effort to more rapidly accumulate information regarding teratogenic risks across a a broad range of anticonvulsants, the North American Antiepileptic Drug Pregnancy Registry (telephone number: 888-233-2334) was recently established. Per the recommendations of the registry's advisory committee, findings from the registry will be released only when information on neonatal outcome has been collected on more than 300 monotherapy exposures, since this is the number of outcomes needed to detect a two- to threefold increase in major birth defects. Thus far, information on the newer anticonvulsants has not yet been released, but it is hoped that with the establishment of such a registry, information about the safety of anticonvulsants for pregnancy can be collected relatively expeditiously. With few data supporting the reproductive safety of these newer anticonvulsants, it is difficult at this time to justify their use during pregnancy, and it is perhaps more prudent to use medications for which teratogenic risks are known as opposed to unknown.

Antipsychotic Agents

While an early case report describing limb malformations raised concerns about first-trimester exposure to haloperidol (Kopelman et al. 1975), recent studies have not demonstrated teratogenic risk associated with older, standard typical neuroleptics of high or low potency (Milkovich and Van den Berg 1976; Slone et al. 1977; van Waes and van de Velde 1969; Waldman and Safferman 1993). However, a meta-analysis of the available studies noted an elevated risk of congenital malformations following first-trimester exposure to low-potency neuroleptics (Altshuler et al. 1996). In clinical practice, higher-potency neuroleptic agents such as fluphenazine, haloperidol, perphenazine, and trifluoperazine may be preferable to low-potency agents or the newer atypical antipsychotics for use in pregnancy (Altshuler et al. 1996).

Information on the reproductive safety of atypical neuroleptic medications remains much more sparse. No adequate human studies are yet available to indicate risk of teratogenicity of clozapine, olanzapine, risperidone, quetiapine, or ziprasidone. To date, there are five published case reports of pregnant women maintained on clozapine during pregnancy, with no evidence of major congenital malformation (Barnas et al. 1994; Dickson and Hogg 1998; Karakula et al. 2004; Stoner et al. 1997; Waldman and Safferman 1993). In addition, the manufacturer of Clozaril has collected outcome information on babies exposed to clozapine (Novartis, personal communication, 1998). Of the 29 exposed neonates, 25 were noted to be healthy, while 4 (13.8%) showed one or more problems, including neonatal convulsions, Turner's syndrome, collarbone fracture, facial deformity, congenital hip dislocation, and blindness. However, the significance of these findings—specifically, as evidence of teratogenic actions of clozapine—remains unclear. More recently, the manufacturer of olanzapine established a registry to collect information on fetal outcomes following prenatal exposure to this drug (Ernst and Goldberg 2002; Goldstein et al. 2000). Outcome data for 96 prospectively reported cases showed

1 case of a major malformation (1%) and an additional 7 cases of perinatal complications (7%). While these findings do not suggest an increased risk in major malformations above the baseline risk, larger sample sizes are needed for more definitive conclusions about teratogenic risks of atypical antipsychotics.

Several case reports have documented transient extrapyramidal symptoms (e.g., motor restlessness, tremor, hypertonicity, dystonic movements, and parkinsonism) in neonates exposed to neuroleptic drugs in utero (Auerbach et al. 1992; Hill et al. 1966; Levy and Wisniewski 1974). These problems have typically been of short duration, and infants exposed to neuroleptic medications in utero were noted to have normal motor development (Desmond et al. 1967). Risks of potential neurobehavioral or cognitive effects of prenatal exposure to older antipsychotic agents have also been considered, but the available data remain very limited and inconclusive. Limited data are available on the long-term neurobehavioral effects of prenatal exposure to antipsychotic agents. An early longitudinal study of estimated IQ and behavior of children exposed to low-potency neuroleptics in utero found no evidence of dysfunction or developmental delays up to age 5 years (Slone et al. 1977).

Treatment Planning for the Pregnant Patient With Bipolar Disorder

Only recently has attention focused on the treatment of BD during pregnancy (Viguera and Cohen 1998; Viguera et al. 2000). Management of BD in the pregnant patient is very challenging, particularly since there are risks associated both with treatment with mood stabilizers and with no treatment, and these various risks have not been fully examined or quantified in pregnancy, thus forcing the patient and physician to make treatment decisions based on partially defined risks. Sound decisions about the continuation or initiation of a psychotropic medication during pregnancy require consideration of the following factors: 1) estimated risk of fetal exposure to medication; 2) substantial risks to the patient, fetus, and family of untreated psychiatric illness in the mother; and 3) typically high risk of relapse associated with discontinuation of maintenance treatment. A discussion of each of these areas should be carried out with the patient and her partner, ideally on more than one occasion before and after conception, with ongoing communication with the patient's obstetrician—all of which should be documented in the patient's medical record. Planning for pregnancy while the patient is euthymic and clinically stable for a prolonged period provides for thoughtful treatment choices and avoids the tendency to precipitously change treatment during an unplanned pregnancy.

Close clinical monitoring during pregnancy is essential. In fact, it may be helpful to model one's clinic approach on how obstetricians care for patients whose pregnancies are considered "high risk" because of the presence of certain medical conditions. Even if all medications are discontinued and there is no need for medication management, the pregnancy of a woman with BD should be considered high risk. Pregnant women with BD are at high risk for relapse during pregnancy and postpartum, and early detection of illness with rapid intervention may significantly reduce morbidity.

Factors That Influence Clinical Decision Making

The most important factors influencing clinical treatment planning during pregnancy are illness history and the estimated safety of specific clinical interventions (pharmacologic or nonpharmacologic). Specific considerations include previous frequency and severity of illness, past and current levels of functioning or impairment, duration of clinical stability with and without medication in the past, known prodromal symptoms that have been characteristic of an impending relapse, history of discontinuation attempts, and time to relapse, as well as average time to recovery from an episode following reintroduction of treatment. During the assessment process, it is useful to inventory previous medication trials and medication responses so as to guide selection of the most effective and safest treatment options in order to minimize fetal exposure. While the newer agents may present an attractive alternative to more conventional therapies, pregnancy is not an appropriate time to experiment with newer agents or use complex drug combinations when simpler and better-known options are available and have proven safe and effective in the past.

Treatment Options

Treatment of BD during pregnancy and the postpartum period is a dynamic process, with decisions about treatment options evolving, depending on the individual patient's course during pregnancy. Each phase represents a distinct time of variable risk for new onset or relapse of illness (Viguera et al. 2000). Use of medications may have a specific set of clinical implications, depending on whether the patient is pregnant, in the postpartum period, or breast-feeding.

The most appropriate treatment algorithm depends on the severity of illness. Patients with a single episode of mania and prompt and full recovery with sustained well-being may tolerate gradual discontinuation of mood stabilizer over at least several weeks before attempting to conceive (Viguera and Cohen 1998; Viguera et al. 2000). In the past, abrupt discontinuation of lithium or other treatments was a common practice, probably largely driven by relatively unbalanced concern about avoidance of liability associated with fetal exposure to a known teratogen. A more appropriate approach is to take a broader view of risks, including risks of recurrent illness in the setting of medication discontinuation. Given the recent data indicating that discontinuation of maintenance pharmacologic treatment is associated with high rates of relapse, especially if it is done abruptly, the taper should be carried out gradually (Baldessarini et al. 1997). The clinical maxim "slower is better" applies here, because there is no standard definition of *gradual* other than a minimum period of greater than 2 weeks. A pregravid trial of medication taper allows both clinician and patient to assess clinical status during taper and during a time when the patient is not taking any medication. At any signs of early relapse, the mood stabilizer can be reintroduced. Plans for continued treatment without a mood stabilizer during pregnancy should then be reevaluated in light of this trial.

Women with BD who have histories of multiple and frequent episodes present a greater challenge, for which there are several options. Some patients may choose to discontinue a mood stabilizer gradually prior to conception. If patients fail this discontinuation trial and become symptomatic during the taper, lithium or another mood stabilizer may be easily resumed, and the feasibility of conceiving while not taking medication should be reassessed. An alternative strategy is to continue maintenance mood stabilizer until the pregnancy is verified. Home pregnancy tests are very reliable and can document pregnancy as early as 10 days postconception. In addition to using a home ovulation predictor kit, a patient may be able to time her treatment discontinuation fairly accurately. This strategy minimizes exposure and affords antimanic prophylaxis for the longest period of time while the patient is trying to conceive. Since utero-placental circulation is not established until approximately 2 weeks postconception, the risk of fetal exposure is minimal. Maintenance of mood stabilizer therapy until early documentation of pregnancy may be particularly prudent for older patients, because the time required for them to conceive may be longer than for younger patients. This strategy, however, involves a more abrupt discontinuation (i.e., taper over <2 weeks), and patients may therefore be at heightened risk for relapse (Baldessarini et al. 1996; Faedda et al. 1993; Suppes et al. 1991). With close clinical follow-up, however, patients can be monitored for early signs of relapse, and medications may be reintroduced as needed.

For women who tolerate discontinuation of maintenance treatment, the decision of when to resume treatment requires sound clinical judgment. Some patients and clinicians may prefer to await initial appearance of symptoms before restarting medication; others may prefer to limit risk of major recurrence by restarting treatment after the first trimester of pregnancy. Some preliminary data suggest that pregnant women with BD who remain well throughout pregnancy may have a lower risk of postpartum relapse compared with women who become ill during pregnancy (Nonacs et al. 199).

For women with the most severe forms of BD, maintenance treatment with a mood stabilizer before and during pregnancy may be the most appropriate strategy. Accepting the relatively small absolute increase in teratogenic risk with first-trimester exposure to lithium, for example, may be justified in such situations, because these patients are at highest risk for clinical deterioration if pharmacologic treatment is withdrawn. Relapse of BD during pregnancy is potentially dangerous to both mother and fetus; it may require aggressive treatment that includes hospitalization as well as exposure to multiple psychotropics at higher dosages. Thus, an informed decision to assume a small amount of quantifiable risk associated with fetal exposure to a medication like lithium may be preferable to the risk of relapse and more intense pharmacologic treatment.

Treatment Planning for the Patient With Bipolar Disorder in the Postpartum Period

Pregnant women with BD should be clearly informed of the unusually high risk of relapse as they enter the postpartum period. Furthermore, this well-documented high rate of postpartum recurrence underscores the need to consider prophylactic intervention to limit these risks (Bratfos and Haug 1966; Brockington et al. 1981; Davidson and Robertson 1985; Kendell et al. 1987; Klompenhouwer and van Hulst 1991; Reich and Winokur 1970; Viguera et al. 2000). Prophylaxis with a mood stabilizer or neuroleptic should be recommended strongly, especially for patients who did not take medication during the pregnancy.

While the data support reintroducing lithium within 48 hours postdelivery, earlier reintroduction of a mood stabilizer at 36 weeks' gestation may be more prudent, given that adequate serum levels of the medication may be achieved prior to entering a period of high risk. While there are no empirically derived data to suggest an advantage of prophylaxis during one time frame versus another, the disadvantage of earlier intervention at 36 weeks seems particularly modest.

Vigilance is required when clinicians elect to decrease a patient's lithium dose before delivery to avoid toxicity, since reductions in serum lithium concentration (especially from high- to low-serum concentrations) may precipitate relapse (Viguera and Cohen 1998; Lapierre et al. 1980; Rosenbaum et al. 1994). Moreover, reduction may directly precede the period of greatest risk for the patient. In addition, reports linking lithium therapy during pregnancy to neonatal toxicity are extremely rare. Clinically, a reasonable option may be to ensure adequate hydration and follow serial serum levels during labor and delivery, as well as during the first few days postpartum, and adjust the dosage accordingly.

Use of an anticonvulsant or an antipsychotic agent for protection during early postpartum months can also be considered, particularly if lithium treatment has been unsuccessful or poorly tolerated in the past. These options are considered secondary choices, however, since there is no research on their use to prevent postpartum illness in women with BD. Use of antidepressants during pregnancy is also widely considered to be generally safe, although their use without a mood-stabilizing treatment in BD is not recommended.

Conclusion

A decision about what constitutes "reasonable risk" during pregnancy calls for shared information and responsibility but ultimately rests with the informed patient. Repeated discussions of information about risks and benefits of treatment options with the patient and her partner, as well as efforts to coordinate care with the attending obstetrician, are important components of an emerging model aimed at optimizing the clinical care of women with bipolar disorder during pregnancy. Finally, research aimed at defining the various risks of treating women with BD through the reproductive cycle and optimizing that treatment is urgently needed.

References

Abou-Saleh MT, Coppen A: Puerperal affective disorders and response to lithium (letter). Br J Psychiatry 142:539, 1983

Altshuler LL, Cohen LS, Szuba MP, et al: Pharmacologic management of psychiatric illness in pregnancy: dilemmas and guidelines. Am J Psychiatry 153:592–606, 1996

Ananth J: Side effects of fetus and infant of psychotropic drug use during pregnancy. Pharmacopsychiatry 11:246–260, 1976

Auerbach JG, Hans SL, Marcus J, et al: Maternal psychotropic medication and neonatal behavior. Neurotoxicol Teratol 14:399–406, 1992

Austin M-PV: Puerperal affective psychosis: is there a case for lithium prophylaxis? Br J Psychiatry 161:692–694, 1992

Baldessarini RJ, Tondo L, Faedda G, et al: Effects of rate of discontinuing lithium maintenance treatment in bipolar disorders. J Clin Psychiatry 57:441–448, 1996

Baldessarini RJ, Tondo L, Floris G, et al: Reduced morbidity after gradual discontinuation of lithium treatment for bipolar I and II disorders: a replication study. Am J Psychiatry 154:551–553, 1997

Baldessarini RJ, Tondo L, Viguera AC: Discontinuing lithium maintenance treatment in bipolar disorders: risks and implications. Bipolar Disord 1:17–24, 1999

Barnas C, Bergant A, Hummer M, et al: Clozapine concentrations in maternal and fetal plasma, amniotic fluid, and breast milk (letter). Am J Psychiatry 151:945, 1994

Blehar MC: Gender differences in risk factors for mood and anxiety disorders: implications for clinical treatment research. Psychopharmacol Bull 31:687–691, 1995

Blehar MC, DePaulo JR Jr, Gershon ES, et al: Women with bipolar disorder: findings from the NIMH Genetics Initiative Sample. Psychopharmacol Bull 34:239–243, 1998

Bratfos OHJ, Haug JO: Puerperal mental disorders in manic-depressive females. Acta Psychiatr Scand 42:285–294, 1966

Briggs GG, Freeman RK, Sumner JY: Drugs in Pregnancy and Lactation. Baltimore, MD, Williams & Wilkins, 1998

Brockington IF, Cernik KF, Schofield EM, et al: Puerperal psychosis: phenomena and diagnosis. Arch Gen Psychiatry 38:829–833, 1981

Brockington IF, Perris C, Kendell RE, et al: The course and outcome of cycloid psychosis. Psychol Med 12:97–105, 1982

Chambers C, Johnson K, Dick L, et al: Birth outcomes in pregnant women taking fluoxetine. N Engl J Med 335:1010–1015, 1996

Clayton-Smith J, Donnai DL: Fetal valproate syndrome. J Med Genet 32:724–727, 1995

Cohen LS, Altshuler L: Pharmacologic management of psychiatric illness during pregnancy and the postpartum period, in The Psychiatric Clinics of North America Annual of Drug Therapy. Edited by Dunner D, Rosenbaum J. Philadelphia, PA, WB Saunders, 1997, pp 21–60

Cohen LS, Friedman JM, Jefferson JW, et al: A reevaluation of risk of in utero exposure to lithium. JAMA 271:146–150, 1994

Cohen LS, Sichel DA, Robertson LM, et al: Postpartum prophylaxis for women with bipolar disorder. Am J Psychiatry 152:1641–1645, 1995

Coryell W, Scheftner WA, Keller M, et al: The enduring psychosocial consequences of mania and depression. Am J Psychiatry 150:720–727, 1993

Davidson J, Robertson E: A follow-up study of postpartum illness. Acta Psychiatr Scand 71:451–457, 1985

Desmond MM, Rudolph AJ, Hill RM: Behavioral alterations in infants born to mothers on psychoactive medication during pregnancy, in Congenital Mental Retardation. Edited by Farrell G. Austin, University of Texas Press, 1967

Dickson R, Hogg L: Pregnancy of a patient treated with clozapine services. Psychiatr Serv 49:1081–1083, 1998

Dion GL, Tohen M, Anthony WA, et al: Symptoms and functioning of patients with bipolar disorder six months after hospitalization. Hosp Community Psychiatry 39:652–657, 1988

D'Orban PT: Women who kill their children. Br J Psychiatry 134:560–571, 1979

Edmonds LD, Oakley GP: Ebstein's anomaly and maternal lithium exposure during pregnancy. Teratology 41:551–552, 1990

Ernst CL, Goldberg JF: The reproductive safety profile of mood stabilizers, atypical antipsychoatics, and broad-spectrum psychotropics. J Clin Psychiatry 63:42–55, 2002

Fabro SE: Clinical Obstetrics. New York, Wiley, 1987

Faedda GL, Tondo L, Baldessarini RJ, et al: Outcome after rapid vs gradual discontinuation of lithium treatment in bipolar disorders. Arch Gen Psychiatry 50:448–455, 1993

Finnerty M, Levin Z, Miller LJ: Acute manic episodes in pregnancy. Am J Psychiatry 153:261–263, 1996

Freeman MP, Wosnitzer Smith K, Freeman S, et al: The impact of reproductive events on the course of bipolar disorder in women. J Clin Psychiatry 63:284–287, 2002

Gitlin MJ, Swendsen J, Heller TL, et al: Relapse and impairment in bipolar disorder. Am J Psychiatry 152:1635–1640, 1995

Goldstein DJ, Corbin LA, Fung MC: Olanzapine-exposed pregnancies and lactation: early experience. J Clin Psychopharmacol 20:399–403, 2000

Goodwin FK, Jamison K: Manic-Depressive Illness. New York, Oxford University Press, 1990

Grof P, Robbins W, Alda M, et al: Protective effect of pregnancy in women with lithium-responsive bipolar disorder. J Affect Disord 61:31–39, 2000

Hill RM, Desmond MM, Kay JL: Extrapyramidal dysfunction in an infant of a schizophrenic mother. J Pediatr 69:589–595, 1966

Holmes LB: The teratogenic effects of anticonvulsant monotherapy: phenobarbital (Pb), carbamazepine (CBZ), and phenytoin (PHT). Teratology 41:565, 1990

Holmes LB, Harvey EA, Coull BA, et al: The teratogenicity of anticonvulsant drugs. N Engl J Med 344:1132–1138, 2001

Jacobson SJ, Jones K, Johnson K, et al: Prospective multicentre study of pregnancy outcome after lithium exposure during first trimester. Lancet 339:530–533, 1992

Jones KL, Lacro RV, Johnson KA, et al: Pattern of malformations in the children of women treated with carbamazepine during pregnancy. N Engl J Med 320:1661–1666, 1989

Kallen B, Tandberg A: Lithium and pregnancy: aA cohort study on manic-depressive women. Acta Psychiatr Scand 68:134–139, 1983

Karakula H, Szajer K, Rpila B, et al: Clozapine and pregnancy—a case history. Pharmacopsychiatry 37:303–304, 2004

Kendell RE, Chalmers JC, Platz C: Epidemiology of puerperal psychoses. Br J Psychiatry 150:662–673, 1987

Kessler RC, McGonagle KA, Zhao S, et al: Lifetime and 12-month prevalence of DSM-III-R psychiatric disorders in the United States: results from the National Comorbidity Survey. Arch Gen Psychiatry 51:8–19, 1994

Klompenhouwer J, van Hulst A: Classification of postpartum psychosis: a study of 250 mother and baby admissions in the Netherlands. Acta Psychiatr Scand 84:255–261, 1991

Kopelman AE, McCullar FW, Heggeness L: Limb malformations following maternal use of haloperidol. JAMA 231:62–64, 1975

Kraepelin E: Manic-Depressive Insanity and Paranoia. Edinburgh, E & S Livingstone, 1921

Lammer EJ, Sever LE, Oakley GP: Teratogen update: valproic acid. Teratology 35:465–473, 1987

Lamotrigine Pregnancy Registry: Interim Report. September 1, 1992 through March 31, 2001. Research Triangle Park, NC, GlaxoSmithKline, 2001

Lapierre YD, Gagnon A, Kokkinidis L: Rapid recurrence of mania following lithium withdrawal. Biol Psychiatry 15:859–864, 1980

Levy W, Wisniewski K: Chlorpromazine causing extrapyramidal dysfunction in newborn infants of psychotic mothers. N Y State J Med 74:684–685, 1974

Lier L, Kastrup M, Rafaelsen O: Psychiatric illness in relation to pregnancy and childbirth, II: diagnostic profiles, psychosocial and perinatal aspects. Nord Psykiatr Tidsskr 43:535–542, 1989

Lindhout D, Meinardi H: Spina bifida and in utero exposure to valproate. Lancet 2:396, 1984

Lindhout D, Omtzigt JG: Teratogenic effects of antiepiletic drugs: implications for the management of epilepsy in women of childbearing
age. Epilepsia 35 (suppl 4):S19–S28, 1994

McNeil TF, Kaij L, Malmquist-Larsson A: Women with nonorganic psychosis: factors associated with pregnancy's effect on mental health.
Acta Psychiatr Scand 70:209–219, 1984

Milkovich L, Van den Berg BJ: An evaluation of the teratogenicity of certain antinauseant drugs. Am J Obstet Gynecol 125:244–248, 1976

Moore KL, Persaud TVN: The Developing Human: Clinically Oriented
Embryology, 7th Edition. Philadelphia, PA, WB Saunders, 2003

Murrow JI, Craig JJ, Russell AJC, et al: Epilepsy and pregnancy: a prospective register in the United Kingdom. J Neurol Sci 187 (suppl 1):
S299, 2001

Nakane Y, Okuma T, Takahashi R, et al: Multi-institutional study on the
teratogenicity and fetal toxicity of antiepileptic drugs: a report of a
collaborative study group in Japan. Epilepsia 21:663–680, 1980

Nonacs R, Viguera AC, Cohen LS: Postpartum course of bipolar illness.
Presentation at the 152nd annual meeting of the American Psychiatric Association, Washington, DC, May 15–20, 1999

Nora JJ, Nora AH, Toews WH: Lithium, Ebstein's anomaly and other
congenital heart defects. Lancet 2(7880):594–595, 1974

Northrup H, Volcik KA: Spina bifida and other neural tube defects.
Curr Probl Pediatr 30:313–332, 2000

Nott PN: Psychiatric illness following childbirth in Southhampton: a
case register study. Psychol Med 12:557–561, 1982

Nulman I, Rovet J, Stewart D, et al: Neurodevelopment of children exposed in utero to antidepressant drugs. N Engl J Med 336:258–262, 1997

Omtzigt JG, Los FJ, Grobbee DE, et al: The risk of spina bifida aperta after first-trimester exposure to valproate in a prenatal cohort. Neurol-
ogy 42:119–125, 1992

Pastuszak A, Schick-Boschetto B, Zuber C, et al: Pregnancy outcome following first-trimester exposure to fluoxetine (Prozac). JAMA
269:2246–2248, 1993

Platz C, Kendell RE: A matched control follow-up and family study of
"puerperal psychosis." Br J Psychiatry 153:90–94, 1988

Pugh TF, Jerath BK, Schmidt WM, et al: Rates of mental disease related
to childbearing. N Engl J Med 268:1224–1228, 1963

Reich T, Winokur G: Postpartum psychosis in patients with manic depressive disease. J Nerv Ment Dis 151:60–68, 1970

Reinisch JM, Sanders SA, Mortensen EL, et al: In utero exposure to phenobarbital and intelligence deficits in adult men. JAMA 274:1518–1525, 1995

Rhode A, Marneros A: Bipolar disorders during pregnancy, post partum, and in menopause, in Bipolar Disorders: 100 Years After Manic-Depressive Insanity. Edited by Marneros A, Angst J. London, Kluwer Academic, 2000, pp 127–137

Robert E, Guibaud P: Maternal valproic acid and congenital neural tube defects. Lancet 2:934, 1982

Rosa FW: Spina bifida in infants of women treated with carbamazepine during pregnancy. N Engl J Med 324:674–677, 1991

Rosenbaum JF, Sachs GS, Lafer B, et al: High rates of relapse in bipolar patients abruptly changed from standard to low serum lithium levels in a double-blind trial. Paper presented at the annual meeting of the American College of Neuropsychopharmacology, San Juan, Puerto Rico, 1994

Sadler T: Langman's Medical Embryology, With Simbryo CD-ROM, 9th Edition. Baltimore, MD, Lippincott Williams & Wilkins, 2003

Schou M: What happened later to the lithium babies: a follow-up study of children born without malformations. Acta Psychiatr Scand 54:193–197, 1976

Schou M, Amdisen A: Lithium and the placenta (letter). Am J Obstet Gynecol 122:541, 1975

Scolnik D, Nulman I, Rovet J, et al: Neurodevelopment of children exposed in utero to phenytoin and carbamazepine monotherapy. JAMA 271:767–770, 1994

Sharma V, Persad P: Effect of pregnancy on three patients with bipolar disorder. Ann Clin Psychiatry 7:39–42, 1995

Slone D, Siskind V, Heinonen OP, et al: Antenatal exposure to the phenothiazines in relation to congenital malformations, perinatal mortality rate, birth weight, and intelligence quotient score. Am J Obstet Gynecol 128:486–488, 1977

Stewart DE: Prophylactic lithium in postpartum affective psychosis. J Nerv Ment Dis 176:485–489, 1988

Stewart DE, Klompenhouwer JL, Kendell RE, et al: Prophylactic lithium in puerperal psychosis: the experience of three centers. Br J Psychiatry 158:393–397, 1991

Stoner S, Sommi R, Marken P, et al: Clozapine use in two full-term pregnancies (letter). J Clin Psychiatry 58:364–365, 1997

Strakowski SM, Williams JR, Fleck DE, et al: Eight-month functional outcome from mania following a first psychiatric hospitalization. J Psychiatr Res 34:193–200, 2000

Suppes T, Baldessarini RJ, Faedda GL, et al: Risk of recurrence following discontinuation of lithium treatment in bipolar disorder. Arch Gen Psychiatry 48:1082–1088, 1991

Suppes T, Baldessarini RJ, Faedda GL, et al: Discontinuation of maintenance treatment in bipolar disorder: risks and implications. Harv Rev Psychiatry 1:131–144, 1993

Targum SD, Davenport YB, Webster MJ: Postpartum mania in bipolar manic-depressive patients withdrawn from lithium carbonate. J Nerv Ment Dis 167:572–574, 1979

Terp IM: Clinical diagnoses and relative risk of admission after parturition. Br J Psychiatry 172:521–528, 1998

van Gent EM, Verhoeven WM: Bipolar illness, lithium prophylaxis, and pregnancy. Pharmacopsychiatry 25:187–191, 1992

van Waes A, van de Velde E: Safety evaluation of haloperidol in the treatment of hyperemesis gravidum. J Clin Psychopharmacol 9:224–227, 1969

Viguera AC, Cohen LS: The course and management of bipolar disorder during pregnancy. Psychopharmacol Bull 34:339–346, 1998

Viguera AC, Nonacs R, Cohen LS, et al: Risk of recurrence of bipolar disorder in pregnant and nonpregnant women after discontinuing lithium maintenance. Am J Psychiatry 157:179–184, 2000

Viguera AC, Cohen LS, Bouffard S, et al: Reproductive decisions by women with bipolar disorder after prepregnancy psychiatric consultation. Am J Psychiatry 159:2102–2104, 2002a

Viguera AC, Cohen LS, Tondo L, et al: Protective effect of pregnancy on the course of lithium-responsive bipolar I disorder. J Affect Disord 72:107–108, 103–105 [author reply], 2002b

Waldman M, Safferman A: Pregnancy and clozapine. Am J Psychiatry 150:168–169, 1993

Weinstein MR, Goldfield MD: Cardiovascular malformations with lithium use during pregnancy. Am J Psychiatry 132:529–531, 1975

Wisner K: Prevention of postpartum episodes in bipolar women. Paper presented at the 151th annual meeting of the American Psychiatric Association, Toronto, ON, Canada, May 1998

Woody J, London W, Wilbanks G: Lithium toxicity in a newborn. Pediatrics 47:94–96, 1971

Zalstein E, Koren G, Einarson T, et al: A case control study on the association between first-trimester exposure to lithium and Ebstein's anomaly. Am J Cardiol 65:817, 1990

Chapter 4

Postpartum Mood Disorders

Ruta M. Nonacs, M.D., Ph.D.

The postpartum period has clearly been defined as a time of increased vulnerability to psychiatric illness in women. In one of the most frequently cited studies of postpartum psychiatric illness, Kendell and colleagues (1987) demonstrated that women experience a dramatic increase in their risk of severe psychiatric illness in the first 3 months after the birth of a child. During the postpartum period, up to 85% of women experience some type of mood disturbance (Henshaw 2003). Most of these women experience the transient and relatively mild mood symptoms called "the blues." About 10%–15% of women experience a more disabling and persistent form of mood disturbance, either postpartum depression (PPD) or postpartum psychosis (G.L. Cooper 1989; P.J. Cooper et al. 1988; Cox et al. 1993). Although postpartum mood disorders are relatively common, depressive symptoms emerging during the postpartum period are frequently overlooked by patients and their caregivers (Coates et al. 2004; Evins et al. 2000). Puerperal affective illness places both the mother and infant at risk and has been associated with significant long-term effects on child development and well-being (Murray and Cooper 1996). Therefore, prompt recognition and treatment of puerperal mood disorders are essential.

Although postpartum psychiatric illness was initially conceptualized as a group of disorders specifically related to childbirth and therefore diagnostically distinct from other types of psychiatric illness, more recent evidence suggests that affective illness emerging during the postpartum period is clinically indistinguishable from affective illness occurring at other times during a woman's life (Frank et al. 1987; O'Hara et al. 1990). Most women with postpartum illness will go on to have mood episodes that are not related to either pregnancy or childbirth.

Postpartum (or puerperal) psychiatric illness is typically divided into three categories: 1) postpartum "blues," 2) postpartum depression, and 3) postpartum psychosis (Table 4–1). Because these three diagnostic subtypes significantly overlap, it is not clear whether they actually represent three distinct disorders. It may be more useful to conceptualize these subtypes as existing along a continuum, where postpartum blues is the mildest and postpartum psychosis the most severe form of puerperal psychiatric illness.

Table 4–1. Classification of postpartum mood disorders

	Incidence	Onset	Characteristic symptoms
Postpartum "blues"	50%–85%	Within first week	Fluctuating mood, tearfulness, anxiety
Postpartum depression	10%–15%	Usually insidious, within first 3 months	Depressed mood, excessive anxiety, insomnia
Puerperal psychosis	0.1%–0.2%	Dramatic, within first 2 weeks	Agitation and irritability, depressed or elated mood, delusions, disorganized behavior

Postpartum psychiatric disorders have not been listed separately in recent revisions of the *Diagnostic and Statistical Manual of Mental Disorders* (DSM-III-R [American Psychiatric Association 1987], DSM-IV [American Psychiatric Association 1994], DSM-IV-TR [American Psychiatric Association 2000]), and no specific criteria for the diagnosis of postpartum psychiatric illness have been provided. According to DSM-IV-TR, postpartum psychiatric illnesses may be indicated with a postpartum onset specifier. The specifier "with postpartum onset" may be used to describe a depressive, manic, or mixed episode of major depressive disorder or bipolar disorder or a brief psychotic disorder, when the episode occurs within the first 4 weeks after delivery.

Although DSM-IV-TR defines *postpartum psychiatric illness* as an affective episode that has its onset within the first 4 weeks after delivery, other authors have described a broader period of risk for the onset of puerperal illness. Risk of postpartum psychiatric illness is the highest in the first month after childbirth; however, several different studies have indicated that women remain at very high risk for affective illness during the first 3 months after delivery (Kendell et al. 1987; O'Hara 1995), and women remain at heightened risk up until 1 year after delivery (Kendell et al. 1987). Thus, the Marcé Society, an international organization dedicated to the study of postpartum psychiatric disorders, defines postpartum psychiatric illness as any episode occurring within the first year after childbirth.

Clinical Features

Postpartum Blues

During the first week after the birth of a child, many women experience a brief period of affective instability, commonly referred to as *postpartum blues* or the "baby blues." Depending on the criteria used to diagnose the blues, it appears that about 50%–85% of women experience the blues (Kennerly and Gath 1989; Pitt 1973). Given the high prevalence of this type of mood disturbance, it may be more accurate to consider the blues a normal experience associated with childbirth rather than a psychiatric disorder. Women with postpartum blues report a variety of symptoms, including a rapidly fluctuating mood, tearfulness, irritability, and anxiety (Kennerly and Gath 1989). These symptoms typically peak on the fourth or fifth day after delivery and may last for a few hours or a few days, remitting spontaneously within 2 weeks of delivery. However, some women with more severe blues may go on to develop PPD (Beck 1996; Henshaw et al. 2004).

Postpartum Depression

During the postpartum period, 10%–15% of women will present with more significant depressive symptoms, or PPD (P.J. Cooper et al. 1988; Cox et al. 1993; Kumar and Robson 1984; O'Hara et al. 1984). In contrast to postpartum blues, PPD is more pervasive and may significantly interfere with a mother's ability to function and to care for her child. Depression most commonly develops insidiously during the first 1–3 postpartum months, although some women report the acute onset of symptoms shortly after childbirth (P.J. Cooper et al. 1988). A significant subpopulation of women actually experience the onset of depressive symptoms *during* pregnancy (Josefsson et al. 2001).

Clinically, PPD is indistinguishable from other types of nonpsychotic major depression. Women typically present with depressed mood, tearfulness, irritability, and loss of interest in their usual activities. Insomnia, fatigue, and loss of appetite are frequently described. Women often express ambivalent or negative feelings toward their infant, and it is common for women with PPD to express doubts or concerns about their ability to care for their children. In its most severe form, PPD may result in profound dysfunction. Suicidal ideation is frequently reported; however, suicide rates appear to be relatively low in women with nonpsychotic major depression (Appleby 1991).

Anxiety symptoms may be prominent in this population, and women may present with generalized anxiety, panic disorder, or hypochondriasis (Hendrick et al. 2000; Ross et al. 2003; Wenzel et al. 2003). In one study, 30% of women diagnosed with PPD also met criteria for an anxiety disorder, most commonly generalized anxiety disorder (Nonacs and Cohen 2001). Although comorbid obsessive-compulsive disorder is not common, women with PPD frequently experience intrusive, obsessive ruminations (Wisner et al. 1999). These obsessions frequently involve the child and often are violent in nature (e.g., thoughts about smothering the infant, dropping the baby down the stairs, or throwing the child out the window). It is important to note that these thoughts are ego-dystonic; women are very distressed by these thoughts and appear to go out of their way to ensure their child's safety. In contrast to patients with postpartum psychosis who may also have thoughts of harming their child, reality testing is intact in these patients.

Postpartum Psychosis

Puerperal psychosis, the most severe form of postpartum psychiatric illness, is a rare event that occurs in about 1–2 per 1,000 women after childbirth (Brockington et al. 1982; Kendell et al. 1987). Its presentation is often dramatic, with onset of symptoms as early as the first 48–72 hours after delivery. The majority of women with puerperal psychosis develop symptoms within the first 2 postpartum weeks (Brockington et al. 1981; Dean and Kendell 1981).

Longitudinal studies indicate that most women with postpartum psychosis have an affective illness, most commonly bipolar disorder (Chaudron and Pies 2003; Dean et al. 1989). The symptoms of puerperal psychosis most closely resemble those of a rapidly evolving manic or mixed episode (Brockington et al. 1981; Dean and Kendell 1981). The earliest signs are restlessness, agitation, irritability, and insomnia. Women with this disorder exhibit a rapidly shifting depressed or elated mood, disorientation or confusion, and disorganized behavior. Delusional beliefs are common and often center on the infant. Commonly reported are delusions that the child is defective or dying, that the infant has special powers, or that the child is either Satan or God. Auditory hallucinations instructing the mother to harm herself or her infant may also occur. Risk of infanticide, as well as of suicide, is high in this population (d'Orban 1979).

Screening for Postpartum Mood Disorders

Despite women having multiple contacts with the medical profession after the birth of a child, postpartum depression frequently goes undiagnosed and untreated (Coates et al. 2004; Evins et al. 2000). Too often, PPD is overlooked or dismissed as a normal or natural consequence of childbirth. One study indicated that although most women with PPD recognized that there was something wrong, only one-third believed that they had depression (Whitton et al. 1996). Complicating the diagnosis of PPD further is that many of the symptoms of depression—for example, disruptions in sleep and appetite, loss of libido, fatigue, and poor concentration—may also occur in nondepressed women after the birth of a child.

Most women with PPD do not report their symptoms to their health care providers (Whitton et al. 1996). Furthermore, it appears that with routine medical care, less than one-third of women with PPD receive any type of intervention (Coates et al. 2004; Evins et al. 2000). Although the symptoms of depression may remit spontaneously, many women are still depressed at 1 year after childbirth in the absence of intervention (Cooper and Murray 1995). Because untreated depression in the mother may have negative effects on the cognitive, emotional, and social development of her child, every effort must be made to facilitate the early detection and treatment of this illness in new mothers.

Although it may be possible to identify certain subpopulations of women at high risk for postpartum mood disturbance (i.e., women with histories of postpartum psychiatric illness) (Beck 1996), it is difficult to predict reliably which women in the general population are likely to develop puerperal illness. Therefore, it is advisable to screen *all* women for depression during the postpartum period. Screening for mood disorders may be somewhat more difficult during this time because many of the neurovegetative signs and symptoms characteristic of major depression (e.g., sleep and appetite disturbance, diminished libido, low energy) are also observed in nondepressed women during the postpartum period; however, certain symptoms, including suicidal ideation, guilt, and anhedonia, may help to distinguish depressed from nondepressed mothers.

The Edinburgh Postnatal Depression Scale (EPDS) is a 10-item, self-rated questionnaire that has been used extensively for the detection of PPD (Cox et al. 1987). On this scale, a score of 12 or greater or an affirmative answer on question 10 (presence of suicidal thoughts) raises concern and indicates a need for more thorough evaluation. Although not commonly employed, the EPDS could easily be integrated into the standard postpartum obstetric visit at 6 weeks, and subsequent pediatric well-baby visits, and can significantly improve the detection of women with postpartum depressive illness (Chaudron et al. 2004; Georgiopoulos et al. 1999).

Course and Prognosis

The duration of postpartum illness appears to be variable. Puerperal episodes are often relatively short-lived and may last no more than 3 months (Cooper and Murray 1995). Many women, however, have a more prolonged illness, and several studies suggest that depressive episodes tend to be longer and more severe in those with histories of major depression (Cooper and Murray 1995; Goodman 2004). Some reports suggest that duration may be related to the severity of illness (Horowitz and Goodman 2004). In general, women with postpartum mood disorders have a good prognosis. In about half of the cases, puerperal depression or psychosis represents the first onset of a recurrent psychiatric illness (O'Hara 1995). Although there appears to be a subpopulation of women who have only puerperal episodes of psychiatric illness, the majority of women with a postpartum affective disorder will go on to have episodes of psychiatric illness unrelated to pregnancy or childbirth (Robling et al. 2000). Rates of recurrent illness are highest among women who experience postpartum psychosis (Garfield et al. 2004); recurrent illness is less likely when the index episode occurred with the first child, when onset was within 1 month of delivery, and in cases of unipolar depression (Robling et al. 2000).

Risk Factors

Demographic Variables

Many groups have investigated the relationship between risk of postpartum psychiatric illness and various demographic variables, including age, marital status, parity, education level, and socioeconomic status (Beck 2001; O'Hara 1995; O'Hara et al. 1984, 1991a; Warner et al. 1996). Most studies have not found a strong association between age and risk for developing puerperal illness; however, there is at least one report of high rates (26%) of PPD among adolescent mothers (Troutman and Cutrona 1990). Although there is little consistent evidence to suggest that any particular demographic variable is a *strong* predictor of puerperal affective illness, a meta-analysis of 84 studies suggests that several demographic variables may be weak predictors of PPD: namely, unwanted or unplanned pregnancy, single status, and lower socioeconomic status (Beck 2001).

Psychosocial Variables

Psychosocial variables appear to play an important role in determining vulnerability to affective illness during the postpartum period. One of the most consistent findings is that among women who report marital dissatisfaction and/or inadequate social supports, postpartum depressive illness is more common (Beck 2001; O'Hara 1986; Paykel et al. 1980; Robertson et al. 2004). Several investigators have also demonstrated that stressful life events occurring either during pregnancy or near the time of delivery appear to increase the likelihood of PPD (Beck 2001; O'Hara 1986; Paykel et al. 1980; Robertson et al. 2004).

History of Affective Disorders

There is a well-defined association between all types of postpartum psychiatric illness and a personal history of affective disorder. At highest risk are women with a history of postpartum psychosis; it is estimated that up to 70% of women who have had one episode of puerperal psychosis will experience another episode following a subsequent pregnancy (Davidson and Robertson 1985; Garfield et al. 2004; Kendell et al. 1987). Similarly, women with histories of PPD are at significant risk, with rates of postpartum recurrence as high as 50% (Garfield et al. 2004). Women with bipolar disorder also appear to be particularly vulnerable during the postpartum period, with rates of postpartum relapse ranging from 30% to 50% (Nonacs et al. 1999; Reich and Winokur 1970; Viguera et al. 2000). This population is also at increased risk of postpartum psychosis (Reich and Winokur 1970). The extent to which a history of unipolar depression influences risk for postpartum illness is less clear. Although studies carried out in the general population suggest a risk of about 24% among women with a history of unipolar depression (O'Hara 1995), a prospective study of a clinical population of women with recurrent major depressive disorder suggested that the risk of postpartum illness may be as high as 50% (Nonacs et al. 2004a).

Depressive Symptoms During Pregnancy

Regardless of illness history, the emergence of depressive symptoms during pregnancy significantly increases the likelihood of PPD, and depression during pregnancy remains one of the most robust predictors of postpartum illness (Beck 2001; O'Hara 1986; O'Hara et al. 1984). One study demonstrated that women who were depressed at 18 weeks of gestation had a threefold greater risk of PPD than women who were euthymic during pregnancy (Heron et al. 2004). For women who were depressed at 32 weeks, the risk was sixfold higher. This study also demonstrated that anxiety during pregnancy significantly increases the risk of PPD.

Impact of Reproductive Hormones on Risk of Illness

The postpartum period is characterized by a rapid shift in the hormonal environment. Within the first 48 hours after delivery, estrogen and progesterone concentrations fall dramatically. Because these gonadal steroids modulate neurotransmitter systems implicated in the pathogenesis of mood disorders, many investigators have proposed a role for these hormones in the emergence of affective illness during the postpartum period. However, there appears to be no consistent correlation between serum levels of estrogen, progesterone, cortisol, or thyroid hormones and the occurrence of postpartum mood disturbance (Hendrick et al. 1998; Wisner and Stowe 1997). Although previous studies indicate that serum levels of gonadal steroids or other hormones may not be useful in identifying women at highest risk for postpartum psychiatric illness, these findings do not exclude a role for reproductive hormones in the etiology of postpartum mood disorders. It has been hypothesized that a subgroup of women may be more sensitive to the hormonal shifts that take place during the postpartum period (as well as similar changes occurring during the premenstrual phase of the menstrual cycle or during the perimenopause) and are more likely to experience clinically significant mood disturbance in response to this change in the hormonal milieu.

Bloch and colleagues (2000) tested this hypothesis by assessing hormonally driven mood changes in a group of women with histories of PPD and a control group of women with no history of affective illness. Both groups were given a gonadotropin-releasing hormone agonist, leuprolide acetate, to shut down ovarian function. Then the women were treated with supraphysiologic levels of estrogen and progesterone for a period of 8 weeks to mimic the hormonal changes that take place during pregnancy. The hormones were abruptly withdrawn in order to simulate the postpartum period. During the withdrawal phase, five of the eight women with histories of PPD developed significant depressive symptoms, similar to those they had experienced during prior episodes of PPD. In contrast, none of the eight women with no history of mood disorder developed mood symptoms during the hormone withdrawal phase. These data suggest that at least some women who develop PPD may be differentially sensitive to changes in the hormonal environment and, when exposed to these changes after delivery, may develop clinically significant depressive symptoms.

Treatment

Psychotherapeutic and Pharmacotherapeutic Interventions

Postpartum Blues

Because postpartum blues are characteristically mild in severity and resolve spontaneously, no specific treatment, other than support and reassurance, is indicated. Although the symptoms may be distressing, they typically do not affect the mother's ability to function and to care for herself or her infant. Psychiatric consultation is generally not required; however, if the symptoms are severe or persist longer than 2 weeks, the patient should be evaluated to rule out the presence of a more significant depressive illness. For women with histories of recurrent affective illness, the blues may herald the development of a more significant PPD (O'Hara et al. 1991b; Paykel et al. 1980).

Postpartum Depression

PPD presents along a continuum. Patients may experience mild or moderate symptoms, or they may present with a more severe depression, characterized by prominent neurovegetative symptoms and marked impairment of functioning. Treatment should be guided by the type and severity of the symptoms and the degree of functional impairment. However, before initiation of psychiatric treatment, medical causes of mood disturbance (e.g., thyroid dysfunction, anemia) must be excluded. Initial evaluation should include a thorough history, physical examination, and routine laboratory tests.

Although PPD is relatively common, few studies have systematically assessed the efficacy of nonpharmacologic and pharmacologic therapies in the treatment of this disorder (for reviews, see Dennis 2004; Dennis and Stewart 2004). There are no data to suggest that PPD should be managed differently from nonpuerperal major depression. Apparently, however, clinicians tend to treat women with PPD with less intensity than they treat nonpuerperal patients. This practice only increases the risk of morbidity in the mother and places her child at risk. Depression that emerges during the postpartum period demands the same intensity of treatment as depression that occurs at other times in a woman's life. As with nonpuerperal depression, earlier initiation of treatment is associated with a better outcome.

For women with mild to moderate depression, nonpharmacologic interventions are often helpful. Furthermore, these types of treatments may be more attractive to women who are breast-feeding and wish to avoid the use of medications. Several preliminary studies have yielded encouraging results for several different types of psychosocial interventions. Given the finding that women who lack adequate social supports appear to be at higher risk for PPD, several groups have explored the use of peer support groups. In one study, 60 women with depressive symptoms at 3 weeks postpartum were recruited and randomly assigned to a peer support group or to standard care (Chen et al. 2000). After 4 weeks, 60% of the women in the support group reported a significant reduction in depressive symptoms, as compared to 33% of the women receiving standard care. Several other studies have demonstrated the positive effects of peer support (Dennis 2003; Morgan et al. 1997); however, not all studies have demonstrated beneficial effects, and it appears that support groups containing both depressed and nondepressed mothers may actually make depressed women feel worse (Fleming et al. 1992).

Several studies have demonstrated that nondirective or supportive counseling administered by health visitors may be effective for treating women with PPD (P.J. Cooper et al. 2003; Holden et al. 1989; Wickberg and Hwang 1996). In the earliest of these studies, 55 women identified as being depressed at 6 weeks postpartum were randomized to receive either eight weekly counseling visits by a health visitor or routine care (Wickberg and Hwang 1996). Of the 26 women in the counseling group who completed the study, 69% recovered fully, as compared to only 39% in the control group.

Several groups have also evaluated the effectiveness of psychotherapy, including cognitive-behavioral therapy (CBT) and interpersonal therapy (IPT), for the treatment of PPD. Appleby and colleagues (1997) randomly assigned 87 women with depressive illness at 6–8 weeks postpartum to one of four treatment groups: 1) fluoxetine plus one CBT session, 2) fluoxetine plus six CBT sessions, (3) placebo plus one CBT session, or 4) placebo plus six CBT sessions. In this study, a significant reduction in depressive symptoms was observed in women after six sessions of CBT delivered over a 12-week period, and CBT (six sessions) was as effective as treatment with fluoxetine in women with PPD. Other studies exploring the use of CBT in smaller samples of women with PPD have also yielded positive results (P.J. Cooper et al. 2003; Honey et al. 2002), and at least one study suggests that CBT may also be effective when used in a group setting (Meager and Milgrom 1996).

IPT has also been shown to be effective for the treatment of women with mild to moderate PPD (O'Hara et al. 2000; Stuart and O'Hara 1995). IPT is a time-limited psychotherapy that focuses primarily on interpersonal relationships and may be used to address many issues important to new mothers with PPD, including role transitions, disruption of relationships with the partner and other social supports, and social isolation. In a study by O'Hara and colleagues (2000), depressed postpartum women ($N=120$) were randomly assigned to either 12 sessions of IPT over 12 weeks or to a waiting list. At the end of the study, women who received IPT had significantly lower ratings of depressive symptoms than control subjects; 43.8% of the IPT group but only 13.7% of control subjects showed complete recovery based on their scores on the Beck Depression Inventory (BDI; score of 9 or lower). Sixty percent of the women in the IPT group showed a 50% reduction in BDI scores, compared with 16% in the control group. In addition, women in the IPT group showed significant improvement on other measures of social adjustment, relative to the control subjects. IPT may also be beneficial when performed in a group setting (Klier et al. 2001).

These nonpharmacologic strategies may be particularly attractive to patients who are reluctant to use psychotropic medications (e.g., women who are breast-feeding) or to patients with milder forms of depressive illness. Further investigation is required to determine the efficacy of these modalities of treatment in women with more severe forms of postpartum mood disturbance. Women with more severe illness, as well as those who do not respond to nonpharmacologic interventions, may choose to receive pharmacologic treatment.

To date, only a few studies have systematically assessed the pharmacologic treatment of PPD (Dennis and Stewart 2004); these studies have demonstrated the efficacy of fluoxetine, sertraline, fluvoxamine, paroxetine, venlafaxine, and bupropion (Appleby et al. 1997; Burt et al. 2001; Cohen et al. 2001; Misri et al. 2004; Nonacs et al. 2004b; Stowe et al. 1995). Most of these studies have been open trials and have shown response rates (defined as a ≥50% reduction in Hamilton Rating Scale for Depression score) ranging from 67% to 87%; the only double-blinded, randomized, controlled trial with a placebo control group demonstrated that fluoxetine was more effective than placebo for the treatment of PPD (Appleby et al. 1997). In all these studies, standard antidepressant doses were effective and well tolerated, although it appears that patients with comorbid anxiety may have a less robust response to antidepressants (Hendrick et al. 2000; Nonacs et al. 2004b).

Although it is often recommended that selective serotonin reuptake inhibitors (SSRIs) be used as the first line of treatment, the choice of an antidepressant should be guided by the patient's prior response to antidepressant medication and a given medication's side-effect profile. In women who are breast-feeding, the choice may also be affected by information regarding the safety of these agents in nursing women (see Chapter 5: "Use of Antidepressants and Mood Stabilizers in Breast-Feeding Women"). In general, SSRIs and selective norepinephrine reuptake inhibitors appear to be ideal first-line agents, being nonsedating and well tolerated. These agents may also be particularly useful for women with comorbid anxiety or obsessive symptoms (Cohen et al. 2001). In general, tricyclic antidepressants (TCAs) are less frequently used. Because they tend to be more sedating, they may be appropriate for women who present with prominent sleep disturbance. However, there are some data to suggest that premenopausal women may respond better to SSRIs than to TCAs (Kornstein et al. 2000). Given the frequency with which anxiety symptoms are noted in women with PPD, adjunctive use of a benzodiazepine (e.g., clonazepam, lorazepam) may also be very helpful.

Women who plan to breast-feed must be informed that all psychotropic medications, including antidepressants, are secreted into the breast milk. Concentrations in breast milk appear to vary widely. The amount of medication to which an infant is exposed depends on several factors (Llewellyn and Stowe 1998; reviewed in Chapter 5). The maternal dosage of medication, frequency of dosing, and rate of maternal drug metabolism are factors that affect how much medication is secreted into the breast milk. The amount of medication to which the child is exposed is also influenced by the frequency and timing of the feedings. Data have accumulated regarding the use of various antidepressants, including the TCAs, fluoxetine, sertraline, and paroxetine, in breast-feeding women (for reviews, see Burt et al. 2001; Newport et al. 2002; see also Chapter 5 in this volume). The data thus far have been encouraging and suggest that significant complications related to neonatal exposure to drugs in breast milk appear to be rare. Although less information is available on other antidepressants, there have been no reports of serious adverse events related to exposure to these medications.

In cases of severe PPD, inpatient hospitalization may be required, particularly for patients who are at risk for suicide. In Great Britain, innovative treatment programs involving joint hospitalization of the mother and baby have been successful; however, mother-infant hospital units are much less common in the United States (Wisner et al. 1996). Women with severe postpartum illness should be considered candidates for electroconvulsive therapy. The option is safe and highly effective and thus should be considered early in treatment. In choosing any treatment strategy, it is important to consider the impact of prolonged hospitalization or treatment of the mother on infant development and attachment.

Postpartum Psychosis

Postpartum psychosis is considered a psychiatric emergency that typically requires inpatient treatment. The management of postpartum psychosis remains largely empirical, with few definitive data and no controlled studies to guide treatment. Given the well-established relationship between puerperal psychosis and bipolar disorder (Reich and Winokur 1970; Targum et al. 1979), postpartum psychosis should be treated as an affective psychosis. Acute treatment with a mood stabilizer, in addition to antipsychotic medications, is indicated. Electroconvulsive therapy (often bilateral) is well tolerated and rapidly effective. Failure to treat puerperal psychosis aggressively places both the mother and the infant at increased risk for harm. Rates of infanticide associated with *untreated* puerperal psychosis have been estimated to be as high as 4% (d'Orban 1979).

Although some authors recommend the discontinuation of psychotropic medications soon after the psychosis clears, others clinicians suggest a longer duration of treatment, arguing that women are at risk for recurrent disease. Given the risk of tardive dyskinesia, prolonged exposure to typical antipsychotic agents should be minimized. Atypical antipsychotic agents may be more useful for long-term maintenance therapy. Treatment with a mood stabilizer, however, should extend beyond the resolution of active symptoms to reduce risk of relapse. The appropriate duration of treatment with a mood stabilizer has not been well defined. It has been shown that the majority of patients with puerperal psychosis have bipolar disorder and will go on to have recurrent nonpuerperal episodes of either mania or depression (Robling et al. 2000); therefore, many authors have suggested long-term maintenance treatment with a mood stabilizer in women who have had one episode of puerperal psychosis.

Hormonal Interventions

Some investigators have also explored the role of hormonal interventions in women with postpartum psychiatric illness. Although early reports suggested that progesterone may be helpful for women with PPD (Dalton 1985; Karuppaswamy and Vlies 2003), there are no systematically derived data to support its use in this setting, and some reports suggest that synthetic progesterone may actually exacerbate mood symptoms during the postpartum period (Lawrie et al. 1998).

There is some evidence to suggest that estrogen has beneficial effects in women with postpartum psychiatric illness. Gregoire and colleagues (1996) described the benefit of transdermal estradiol-17β (200 µg daily) in a double-blind, placebo-controlled study of women with PPD. At 12 weeks, 80% of the women receiving estrogen ($n=37$) were no longer depressed (scoring <14 on the EPDS), compared with 31% in the placebo group ($n=24$). Although this study was small and was confounded by the inclusion of patients who were concurrently treated with antidepressant medication, it is the first to demonstrate that estrogen alone (or possibly when used as an adjunct to an antidepressant) may be useful in the treatment of postpartum depression. More recently, Ahokas and colleagues (2001) used sublingual estradiol-17β as monotherapy in an open-label study of 23 women with PPD. In this study, 19 of 23 women experienced recovery after 2 weeks of treatment with estradiol. A similar study from the same group also showed a beneficial effect of estradiol in 10 women with postpartum psychosis (Ahokas et al. 2000).

These studies suggest a role for estrogen in the treatment of women with postpartum psychiatric illness; however, these treatments remain experimental. Estrogen delivered in the acute postpartum period is not without risk and has been associated with changes in breast milk production, as well as more significant, thromboembolic events. Because antidepressants are safe, well tolerated, and highly effective, they remain the first choice for treatment in women with PPD.

Prophylactic Interventions

Although it is difficult to predict reliably which women in the general population will experience psychiatric illness after the birth of a child, it is possible to identify certain subgroups of women (i.e., women with a history of mood disorder) who are more vulnerable to postpartum illness. Given this opportunity to identify certain populations of women at higher risk *before* delivery, several investigators have explored the potential efficacy of prophylactic interventions in these populations of women at highest risk for postpartum affective illness.

Several studies have demonstrated that women with histories of puerperal psychosis benefit from prophylactic treatment with lithium instituted either prior to delivery (at 36 weeks' gestation) or no later than the first 48 hours postpartum (Austin 1992; Stewart 1988; Stewart et al. 1991). Lithium prophylaxis is also effective for women with histories of bipolar disorder; it appears to significantly reduce relapse rates, as well as to diminish the severity and duration of puerperal illness (Cohen et al. 1993; Viguera et al. 2000). In a retrospective study including 27 pregnant women with bipolar disorder, Cohen and colleagues (1993) demonstrated that only 1 of the 14 patients taking lithium prophylaxis relapsed within the first 3 months postpartum, as compared with 8 of the 13 who did not receive prophylaxis. Although the efficacy of lithium in this setting has been described, the efficacy of other mood stabilizers (i.e., valproic acid, carbamazepine) and antipsychotic agents in this setting has not yet been determined. In a nonrandomized clinical trial in which 26 pregnant women with bipolar disorder chose to receive either valproic acid or symptom monitoring (without drug) after delivery, valproic acid was no more effective than monitoring for the prevention of postpartum episodes of bipolar illness, although women treated with valproic acid tended to have less severe symptoms of hypomania or mania (Wisner et al. 2004).

For women with histories of PPD, Wisner and colleagues described a beneficial effect of prophylactic antidepressant administered after delivery (Wisner and Wheeler 1994; Wisner et al. 2004b). In an open-label trial in 23 women with histories of PPD, treatment with either a TCA or an SSRI, administered after delivery, resulted in a reduction in risk of postpartum illness (Wisner and Wheeler 1994). In a subsequent double-blind, placebo-controlled study from the same group, 22 women with histories of postpartum depression were randomly assigned to receive treatment with either sertraline or placebo (Wisner et al. 2004b). Sertraline was introduced on the first postpartum day (on average, within 15 hours of delivery) at a dose of 50 mg per day and increased to 75 mg at week 5. Of the 14 women who received sertraline, only 1 woman had recurrence of depression. In contrast, 4 (50%) of the 8 women in the placebo group developed depressive symptoms. Other studies have not yielded positive results. A randomized, placebo-controlled study from the same group did not demonstrate a positive effect in women treated prophylactically with nortriptyline (Wisner et al. 2001). The authors hypothesized that nortriptyline may be less effective than SSRIs for the prevention and treatment of PPD.

The extent to which this prophylactic intervention may be useful in women with histories of major depressive disorder is not yet clear but is currently under investigation; nonetheless, it is often recommended that women with histories of recurrent depression remain taking an antidepressant throughout the postpartum period to minimize their risk of relapse after delivery (Altshuler et al. 2001).

Psychosocial interventions, such as psychoeducational or support groups, are frequently included in the care of women during the postpartum period. The extent to which these interventions are effective in preventing postpartum mood disturbance is not clear. Several investigators have explored the use of psychoeducational groups during pregnancy and the postpartum period and have demonstrated a significant reduction in the incidence of PPD in women who received this intervention, as compared to untreated control subjects (Cowan and Cowan 1987; Gordon and Gordon 1960; Ogrodniczuk and Piper 2003). Other studies have not yielded positive results (see Hagan et al. 2004; Marks et al. 2003).

In summary, prophylaxis against postpartum depressive illness may be conceptualized along a continuum, on which some women are at lower risk for puerperal illness while others appear to be at higher risk for puerperal decompensation and are candidates for some type of prophylactic intervention. All women, regardless of illness history, should be monitored for mood symptoms during the postpartum period. Women with pregravid histories of a mood or anxiety disorder are clearly at higher risk and should be closely monitored for recurrent symptoms during the postpartum period. Women with histories of recurrent major depression or those who have experienced depressive symptoms during pregnancy may also benefit from antidepressant prophylaxis. Although a less aggressive, "wait and see" approach is appropriate for women with no history of postpartum psychiatric illness, women at highest risk for postpartum affective illness—those with bipolar disorder or histories of postpartum psychiatric illness—deserve not only close monitoring but also specific prophylactic measures.

Conclusion

Postpartum psychiatric illness comprises a highly prevalent group of disorders that affect women during their childbearing years. Although postpartum blues are relatively benign and require no specific intervention, postpartum depression and postpartum psychosis cause significant distress and dysfunction. Despite women's multiple contacts with the medical profession during the postpartum period, puerperal mood disorders are frequently missed and many women go without treatment.

Untreated mood disorder places the mother at risk for recurrent and treatment-refractory illness. Furthermore, a growing body of literature demonstrates the detrimental effect of maternal depression on child development and well-being (Murray and Cooper 1996). Attachment difficulties are common in new mothers and may be quite severe in women with PPD or postpartum psychosis (Cicchetti et al. 1998; Edhborg et al. 2003; Lyons-Ruth et al. 1993). Long-term follow-up studies have shown that behavioral difficulties and cognitive deficits are more common in the children of mothers with PPD (Beck 1998; Cogill et al. 1986; Cummings and Davies 1994; Murray and Cooper 1996, 1997). Studies have also indicated that these children show significant and long-standing difficulties in emotional regulation (Murray et al. 1999). What is particularly concerning is that the effects of maternal depression occurring during the first year of a child's life may be evident long after the episode resolves; Hay and colleagues (2001) demonstrated that the 11-year-old children of women who were depressed at 3 months postpartum had significantly lower IQ scores and were more likely to have attention problems and special educational needs than the children of mothers who were not depressed.

One of the most important objectives is to increase awareness among the spectrum of health care professionals who care for women during pregnancy and the puerperium, so that postpartum mood disorders may be identified early and treated appropriately. Effective pharmacologic and nonpharmacologic therapies are available. For certain subgroups at high risk for puerperal illness, there is also the possibility of effective prophylactic interventions that may limit both maternal and infant morbidity.

References

Ahokas A, Aito M, Rimon R: Positive treatment effect of estradiol in postpartum psychosis: a pilot study. J Clin Psychiatry 61:166–169, 2000

Ahokas A, Kaukoranta J, Wahlbeck K, et al: Estrogen deficiency in severe postpartum depression: successful treatment with sublingual physiologic 17beta-estradiol: a preliminary study. J Clin Psychiatry 62:332–336, 2001

Altshuler LL, Cohen LS, Moline ML, et al: The Expert Consensus Guideline Series. Treatment of depression in women. Postgrad Med (Spec No), March 2001, pp 1–107

American Psychiatric Association: Diagnostic and Statistical Manual of Mental Disorders, 3rd Edition, Revised. Washington, DC, American Psychiatric Association, 1987

American Psychiatric Association: Diagnostic and Statistical Manual of Mental Disorders, 4th Edition. Washington, DC, American Psychiatric Association, 1994

American Psychiatric Association: Diagnostic and Statistical Manual of Mental Disorders, 4th Edition, Text Revision. Washington, DC, American Psychiatric Association, 2000

Appleby L: Suicide during pregnancy and in the first postnatal year. BMJ 302:137–140, 1991

Appleby L, Warner R, Whitton A, et al: A controlled study of fluoxetine and cognitive-behavioral counselling in the treatment of postnatal depression. BMJ 314:932–936, 1997

Austin MP: Puerperal affective psychosis: is there a case for lithium prophylaxis? Br J Psychiatry 161:692–694, 1992

Beck CT: A meta-analysis of predictors of postpartum depression. Nurs Res 45:297–303, 1996

Beck CT: The effects of postpartum depression on child development: a meta-analysis. Arch Psychiatr Nurs 12:12–20, 1998

Beck CT: Predictors of postpartum depression: an update. Nurs Res 50:275–285, 2001

Bloch M, Schmidt PJ, Danaceau M, et al: Effects of gonadal steroids in women with a history of postpartum depression. Am J Psychiatry 157: 924–930, 2000

Brockington IF, Cernik KF, Schofield EM, et al: Puerperal psychosis: phenomena and diagnosis. Arch Gen Psychiatry 38:829–833, 1981

Brockington IF, Winokur G, Dean C: Puerperal psychosis, in Motherhood and Mental Illness. Edited by Brockington IF, Kumar R. London, Academic Press, 1982, pp 37–69

Burt VK, Suri R, Altshuler L, et al: The use of psychotropic medications during breast-feeding. Am J Psychiatry 158:1001–1009, 2001

Chaudron LH, Pies RW: The relationship between postpartum psychosis and bipolar disorder: a review. J Clin Psychiatry 64:1284–1292, 2003

Chaudron LH, Szilagyi PG, Kitzman HJ, et al: Detection of postpartum depressive symptoms by screening at well-child visits. Pediatrics 113: 551–558, 2004

Chen CH, Tseng YF, Chou FH, et al: Effects of support group intervention in postnatally distressed women: a controlled study in Taiwan. J Psychosom Res 49:395–399, 2000

Cicchetti D, Rogosch FA, Toth SL: Maternal depressive disorder and contextual risk: contributions to the development of attachment insecurity and behavior problems in toddlerhood. Dev Psychopathol 10:283–300, 1998

Coates AO, Schaefer CA, Alexander JL: Detection of postpartum depression and anxiety in a large health plan. J Behav Health Serv Res 31:117–133, 2004

Cogill SR, Caplan HL, Alexandra H, et al: Impact of maternal postnatal depression on cognitive development of young children. BMJ (Clin Res Ed) 292:1165–1167, 1986

Cohen LS, Sichel DA, Robertson LM, et al: Postpartum prophylaxis for women with bipolar disorder. Am J Psychiatry 152:1641–1645, 1995

Cohen, LS, Viguera AC, Bouffard SM, et al: Venlafaxine in the treatment of postpartum depression. J Clin Psychiatry 62:592–596, 2001

Cooper GL: The safety of fluoxetine: an update. Br J Psychiatry 153 (suppl 3):77–86, 1989

Cooper PJ, Murray L: Course and recurrence of postnatal depression: evidence for the specificity of the diagnostic concept. Br J Psychiatry 166:191–195, 1995

Cooper PJ, Campbell EA, Day A, et al: Non-psychotic psychiatric disorder after childbirth: a prospective study of prevalence, incidence, course and nature. Br J Psychiatry 152:799–806, 1988

Cooper PJ, Murray L, Wilson A, et al: Controlled trial of the short- and long-term effect of psychological treatment of post-partum depression, I: impact on maternal mood. Br J Psychiatry 182:412–419, 2003

Cowan C, Cowan P: Preventive intervention for couples becoming parents, in Research on Support for Parents and Infants in the Postnatal Period. Edited by Zachariah Boukydis CF. Norwood, NJ, Ablex, 1987, pp 225–233

Cox JL, Holden JM, Sagovsky R: Detection of postnatal depression: development of the 10-item Edinburgh Postnatal Depression Scale. Br J Psychiatry 150:782–786, 1987

Cox JL, Murray D, Chapman G: A controlled study of the onset, duration, and prevalence of postnatal depression. Br J Psychiatry 163:27–31, 1993

Cummings EM, Davies PT: Maternal depression and child development. J Child Psychol Psychiatry 35:73–112, 1994

Dalton K: Progesterone prophylaxis used successfully in postnatal depression. Practitioner 229:507–508, 1985

Davidson J, Robertson E: A follow-up study of postpartum illness. Acta Psychiatr Scand 71:451–457, 1985

Dean C, Kendell RE: The symptomatology of puerperal illness. Br J Psychiatry 139:128–133, 1981

Dean C, Williams RJ, Brockington IF: Is puerperal psychosis the same as bipolar manic-depressive disorder? A family study. Psychol Med 19:637–647, 1989

Dennis CL: The effect of peer support on postpartum depression: a pilot randomized controlled trial. Can J Psychiatry 48:115–124, 2003

Dennis CL: Treatment of postpartum depression, part 2: a critical review of nonbiological interventions. J Clin Psychiatry 65:1252–1265, 2004

Dennis CL, Stewart DE: Treatment of postpartum depression, Part 1: a critical review of biological interventions. J Clin Psychiatry 65:1242–1251, 2004

d'Orban PT: Women who kill their children. Br J Psychiatry 134:560–571, 1979

Edhborg M, Lundh W, Seimyr L, et al: The parent-child relationship in the context of maternal depressive mood. Arch Women Ment Health 6:211–216, 2003

Evins GG, Theofrastous JP, Galvin SL: Postpartum depression: a comparison of screening and routine clinical evaluation. Am J Obstet Gynecol 182:1080–1082, 2000

Fleming AS, Klein E, Corter C: The effects of a social support group on depression, maternal attitudes and behavior in new mothers. J Child Psychol Psychiatry 33:685–698, 1992

Frank E, Kupfer DJ, Jacob M, et al: Pregnancy-related affective episodes among women with recurrent depression. Am J Psychiatry 144:288–293, 1987

Garfield P, Kent A, Paykel ES, et al: Outcome of postpartum disorders: a 10 year follow-up of hospital admissions. Acta Psychiatr Scand 109:434–439, 2004

Georgiopoulos AM, Bryan TL, Yawn BP, et al: Population-based screening for postpartum depression. Obstet Gynecol 93:653–657, 1999

Goodman JH: Postpartum depression beyond the early postpartum period. J Obstet Gynecol Neonatal Nurs 33:410–420, 2004

Gordon R, Gordon K: Social factors in the prevention of postpartum emotional problems. Obstet Gynecol 15:433–438, 1960

Gregoire AJ, Kumar R, Everitt B, et al: Transdermal estrogen for treatment of severe postnatal depression. Lancet 347:930–933, 1996

Hagan R, Evans SF, Pope S: Preventing postnatal depression in mothers of very preterm infants: a randomised controlled trial. BJOG 111:641–647, 2004

Hay DF, Pawlby S, Sharp D, et al: Intellectual problems shown by 11-year-old children whose mothers had postnatal depression. J Child Psychol Psychiatry 42:871–889, 2001

Hendrick V, Altshuler L, Suri R: Hormonal changes in the postpartum and implications for postpartum depression. Psychosomatics 39:93–101, 1998

Hendrick V, Altshuler L, Strouse T, et al: Postpartum and nonpostpartum depression: differences in presentation and response to pharmacologic treatment. Depress Anxiety 11:66–72, 2000

Henshaw C: Mood disturbance in the early puerperium: a review. Arch Women Ment Health 6 (suppl 2):S33–S42, 2003

Henshaw C, Foreman D, Cox J: Postnatal blues: a risk factor for postnatal depression. J Psychosom Obstet Gynaecol 25:267–272, 2004

Heron J, O'Connor TG, Evans J, et al: The course of anxiety and depression through pregnancy and the postpartum in a community sample. J Affect Disord 80:65–73, 2004

Holden JM, Sagovsky R, Cox JL: Counselling in a general practice setting: controlled study of health visitor intervention in treatment of postnatal depression. BMJ 298:223–226, 1989

Honey KL, Bennett P, Morgan M: A brief psycho-educational group intervention for postnatal depression. Br J Clin Psychol 41:405–409, 2002

Horowitz JA, Goodman J: A longitudinal study of maternal postpartum depression symptoms. Res Theory Nurs Pract 18:149–163, 2004

Josefsson A, Berg G, Nordin C, et al: Prevalence of depressive symptoms in late pregnancy and postpartum. Acta Obstet Gynecol Scand 80:251–255, 2001

Karuppaswamy J, Vlies R: The benefit of oestrogens and progestogens in postnatal depression. J Obstet Gynaecol 23:341–346, 2003

Kendell RE, Chalmers JC, Platz C: Epidemiology of puerperal psychoses. Br J Psychiatry 150:662–673, 1987

Kennerley H, Gath D: Maternity blues, I: detection and measurement by questionnaire. Br J Psychiatry 155:356–362, 1989

Klier CM, Muzik M, Rosenblum KL, et al: Interpersonal psychotherapy adapted for the group setting in the treatment of postpartum depression. J Psychother Pract Res 10:124–131, 2001

Kornstein SG, Schatzberg AF, Thase ME, et al: Gender differences in treatment response to sertraline versus imipramine in chronic depression. Am J Psychiatry 157:1445–1452, 2000

Kumar R, Robson KM: A prospective study of emotional disorders in childbearing women. Br J Psychiatry 144:35–47, 1984

Lawrie TA, Hofmeyr GJ, De Jager M, et al: A double-blind randomised placebo controlled trial of postnatal norethisterone enanthate: the effect on postnatal depression and serum hormones. Br J Obstet Gynaecol 105:1082–1090, 1998

Llewellyn A, Stowe ZN: Psychotropic medications in lactation. J Clin Psychiatry 59 (suppl 2):41–52, 1998

Lyons-Ruth K, Alpern L, Repacholi B: Disorganized infant attachment classification and maternal psychosocial problems as predictors of hostile-aggressive behavior in the preschool classroom. Child Dev 64:572–585, 1993

Marks MN, Siddle K, Warwick C: Can we prevent postnatal depression? A randomized controlled trial to assess the effect of continuity of midwifery care on rates of postnatal depression in high-risk women. J Matern Fetal Neonatal Med 13:119–127, 2003

Meager I, Milgrom J: Group treatment for postpartum depression: a pilot study. Aust N Z J Psychiatry 30:852–860, 1996

Misri S, Reebye P, Corral M, et al: The use of paroxetine and cognitive-behavioral therapy in postpartum depression and anxiety: a randomized controlled trial. J Clin Psychiatry 65:1236–1241, 2004

Morgan M, Matthey S, Barnett B, et al: A group programme for postnatally distressed women and their partners. J Adv Nurs 26:913–920, 1997

Murray L, Cooper PJ: The impact of postpartum depression on child development. Int Rev Psychiatry 8:55–63, 1996

Murray L, Cooper PJ: Postpartum depression and child development. Psychol Med 27:253–260, 1997

Murray L, Sinclair D, Cooper P, et al: The socioemotional development of 5-year-old children of postnatally depressed mothers. J Child Psychol Psychiatry 40:1259–1271, 1999

Newport DJ, Hostetter A, Arnold A, et al: The treatment of postpartum depression: minimizing infant exposures. J Clin Psychiatry 63 (suppl 7): 31–44, 2002

Nonacs RM, Cohen LS: Postpartum symptom expression. Presentation at the 154th annual meeting of the American Psychiatric Association, New Orleans, LA, May 5–10, 2001

Nonacs RM, Viguera AC, Cohen LS: Postpartum course of bipolar illness. Presentation at the 152nd annual meeting of the American Psychiatric Association, Washington, DC, May 15–20, 1999

Nonacs RM, Cohen LS, Viguera AC, et al: Risk for recurrent depression during the postpartum period: a prospective study. Presentation at the 157th annual meeting of the American Psychiatric Association, New York City, May 1–6, 2004a

Nonacs RM, Soares CN, Viguera AC, et al: Wellbutrin SR for the treatment of postpartum depression. Presentation at the 157th annual meeting of the American Psychiatric Association, New York City, May 1–6, 2004b

Ogrodniczuk JS, Piper WE: Preventing postnatal depression: a review of research findings. Harv Rev Psychiatry 11:291–307, 2003

O'Hara MW: Social support, life events, and depression during pregnancy and the puerperium. Arch Gen Psychiatry 43:569–573, 1986

O'Hara MW: Postpartum Depression: Causes and Consequences. New York, Springer-Verlag, 1995

O'Hara MW, Neunaber DJ, Zekoski EM: Prospective study of postpartum depression: prevalence, course, and predictive factors. J Abnorm Psychol 93:158–171, 1984

O'Hara MW, Zekoski EM, Philipps LH, et al: Controlled prospective study of postpartum mood disorders: comparison of childbearing and nonchildbearing women. J Abnorm Psychol 99:3–15, 1990

O'Hara MW, Schlechte JA, Lewis DA, et al: Controlled prospective study of postpartum mood disorders: psychological, environmental, and hormonal factors. J Abnorm Psychol 100:63–73, 1991a

O'Hara MW, Schlechte JA, Lewis DA, et al: Prospective study of postpartum blues: biologic and psychosocial factors. Arch Gen Psychiatry 48:801–806, 1991b

O'Hara MW, Stuart S, Gorman LL, et al: Efficacy of interpersonal psychotherapy for postpartum depression. Arch Gen Psychiatry 57:1039–1045, 2000

Paykel ES, Emms EM, Fletcher J: Life events and social support in puerperal depression. Br J Psychiatry 136:339–346, 1980

Pitt B: Maternity blues. Br J Psychiatry 122:431–433, 1973

Reich T, Winokur G: Postpartum psychoses in patients with manic depressive disease. J Nerv Ment Dis 151:60–68, 1970

Robertson E, Grace S, Wallington T, et al: Antenatal risk factors for postpartum depression: a synthesis of recent literature. Gen Hosp Psychiatry 26:289–295, 2004

Robling SA, Paykel ES, Dunn VJ, et al: Long-term outcome of severe puerperal psychiatric illness: a 23 year follow-up study. Psychol Med 30:1263–1271, 2000

Ross LE, Gilbert Evans SE, Sellers EM, et al: Measurement issues in postpartum depression, Part 1: anxiety as a feature of postpartum depression. Arch Women Ment Health 6:51–57, 2003

Stewart DE: Prophylactic lithium in postpartum affective psychosis. J Nerv Ment Dis 176:485–489, 1988

Stewart DE, Klompenhouwer JL, Kendell RE, et al: Prophylactic lithium in puerperal psychosis: the experience of three centers. Br J Psychiatry 158:393–397, 1991

Stowe ZN, Casarella J, Landry J, et al: Sertraline in the treatment of women with postpartum major depression. Depression 3:49–55, 1995

Stuart S, O'Hara MW: Treatment of postpartum depression with interpersonal psychotherapy (letter). Arch Gen Psychiatry 52:75–76, 1995

Targum SD, Davenport YB, Webster MJ: Postpartum mania in bipolar manic depressive patients withdrawn from lithium carbonate. J Nerv Ment Dis 167:572–574, 1979

Troutman BR, Cutrona CE: Nonpsychotic postpartum depression among adolescent mothers. J Abnorm Psychol 99:69–78, 1990

Viguera AC, Nonacs R, Cohen LS, et al: Risk of recurrence of bipolar disorder in pregnant and nonpregnant women after discontinuing lithium maintenance. Am J Psychiatry 157:179–184, 2000

Warner R, Appleby L, Whitton A, et al: Demographic and obstetric risk factors for postnatal psychiatric morbidity. Br J Psychiatry 168:607–611, 1996

Wenzel A, Haugen EN, Jackson LC, et al: Prevalence of generalized anxiety at eight weeks postpartum. Arch Women Ment Health 6:43–49, 2003

Whitton A, Warner R, Appleby L: The pathway to care in post-natal depression: women's attitudes to post-natal depression and its treatment. Br J Gen Pract 46:427–428, 1996

Wickberg B, Hwang CP: Counselling of postnatal depression: a controlled study on a population based Swedish sample. J Affect Disord 39:209–216, 1996

Wisner KL, Stowe ZN: Psychobiology of postpartum mood disorders. Semin Reprod Endocrinol 15:77–89, 1997

Wisner KL, Wheeler SB: Prevention of recurrent postpartum major depression. Hosp Community Psychiatry 45:1191–1196, 1994

Wisner KL, Jennings KD, Conley B: Clinical dilemmas due to the lack of inpatient mother-baby units. Int J Psychiatry Med 26:479–493, 1996

Wisner KL, Peindl KS, Gigliotti T, et al: Obsessions and compulsions in women with postpartum depression. J Clin Psychiatry 60:176–180, 1999

Wisner KL, Perel JM, Peindl KS, et al: Prevention of recurrent postpartum depression: a randomized clinical trial. J Clin Psychiatry 62:82–86, 2001

Wisner KL, Hanusa BH, Peindl KS, et al: Prevention of postpartum episodes in women with bipolar disorder. Biol Psychiatry 56:592–596, 2004a

Wisner KL, Perel JM, Peindl KS, et al: Prevention of postpartum depression: a pilot randomized clinical trial. Am J Psychiatry 161:1290–1292, 2004b

Chapter 5

Use of Antidepressants and Mood Stabilizers in Breast-Feeding Women

Kimberly Ragan, M.S.W.
Zachary N. Stowe, M.D.
D. Jeffrey Newport, M.D., M.S., M.Div.

Since the mid-1980s, breast-feeding has garnered global recognition by virtually all professional organizations as the ideal form of nutrition for infants (Newton 2004). As a result, the proportion of women choosing to breast-feed continues to rise (Ryan et al. 2002), and the duration of breast-feeding has increased (Nichols-Johnson 2004). Despite this universal acceptance of breast-feeding, decisions regarding lactation are complicated by the common occurrence of postnatal maternal illness. Prescribing medications to lactating women presents a clinical conundrum in which infant exposure to mediation must be weighed against the benefits of breast-feeding. Breast-feeding women routinely take prescription medications following childbirth (e.g., opiate analgesics, allergy medications) with limited concern for exposure of the nursing infant. Furthermore, lactating women with chronic medical conditions (e.g., epilepsy, migraine headaches) are increasingly encouraged to use medications for these conditions, and several such medications are now deemed "compatible" with breast-feeding. In contrast, the use of psychotropic medications for the treatment of maternal mental illness has historically been discouraged. This apparent discrepancy gives rise to two important questions:

1. Where does mental illness lie on the spectrum of medical conditions warranting treatment even during lactation?
2. Which factors and/or professional organization guidelines should influence clinical treatment planning?

Although many review articles have focused on psychotropic medications during pregnancy and lactation (Cohen et al. 2004; Hendrick and Altshuler 2002; Newport and Stowe 2003; Newport et al. 2001; Nonacs and Cohen 2003; Spencer et al. 2001; Stowe et al. 2001), seldom have these reviews critically addressed the above questions and others germane to the interpretation and clinical application of the existing data.

In this review, we provide a critical appraisal of literature on the use of antidepressants and mood stabilizers in lactating women, particularly with respect to determining nursing infant exposure. To expand beyond previous reviews, we have included recommendations from the *Physicians' Desk Reference* (PDR) and the American Academy of Pediatrics Committee on Breast Feeding (AAP).

Pharmacologic Treatment Options for Unipolar Depression and Bipolar Disorder in Breast-Feeding

A *MEDLINE* search identified 148 original research reports for the use of antidepressants or mood stabilizers during breast-feeding. With few exceptions, the parent compound and/or metabolites were found in human breast milk; thus, the nursing infant is always exposed to medication. To afford a detailed characterization of infant exposure and provide a basis for comparing individual medications, investigators have typically emphasized either breast milk concentration or the nursing infant's serum concentration.

Historically, the de facto standard for breast-feeding safety has been defined as an estimated infant daily dose (estimated from the milk/plasma [M/P] ratio and infant weight) of less than 10% of the maternal daily dose. This standard has essentially no scientific justification. Conclusions based on such measures are laden with potential confounds. For example, the M/P ratio often is determined at a single time point that fails to account for any time-post-dose effects or foremilk-to-hindmilk concentration gradient. Our group (Stowe et al. 1997, 2000), in collaboration with others (Suri et al. 2002), has clearly demonstrated that antidepressant excretion into breast milk varies from the first portion of breast milk (foremilk) to the latter portion (hindmilk) for sertraline, paroxetine, and fluoxetine. Similarly, the excretion into human breast milk varies with time post dose. Therefore, accurate estimation of infant dose from M/P ratios based on spot breast milk sampling is unlikely. In addition, the use of infant weight assumes that for a given weight, the infant will have a similar volume of distribution compared with the mother. A recent study with fluoxetine (Suri et al. 2002) confirmed the limited utility of M/P ratios. In this study, the estimated infant daily dose was calculated by three methods: 1) M/P ratio and infant weight; 2) 24-hour total collection of breast milk; and 3) mathematical modeling using gradient and time course calculations. The mathematical model was the strongest predictor of nursing infant serum concentrations, supporting the utility of such detailed investigations in determining infant exposure.

The emerging standard for quantifying nursing infant exposure is the measurement of nursing infant serum concentrations. This measure may be more reliable than previous methods of comparison, as potential confounds such as gastrointestinal absorption and infant metabolic capacity are eliminated. However, other confounds limit the use of infant serum concentrations to make definitive comparisons between medications:

1. Nursing infant serum concentrations, even in the research setting, are often below the limit of detection for a given assay. Clinical laboratory assays are even less likely to detect measurable quantities in the concentration range typically encountered in nursing infants. Research assays with confirmed detection limits are required but are not always available.
2. Nursing infant serum concentrations typically represent the total concentration and do not distinguish between the "free" and "bound" compound. Only the "free" portion is available for

entry into the central nervous system (CNS), and some medications (e.g., valproate) demonstrate concentration-dependent binding.

3. Nursing infant serum concentrations are not typically reported in molar concentrations, and different medications have very different binding affinities or even distinct modes of action. For example, the binding affinity of paroxetine for the serotonin transporter is more than 20 times greater than that of fluoxetine, 10 times greater than that of citalopram, and 4 times greater than that of sertraline (Owens et al. 1997).

4. The correlation between serum concentrations and CNS concentrations for the majority of medications is yet to be confirmed.

In summary, use of infant serum concentrations has advantages over reliance on breast milk concentrations and the M/P ratio as a measure of infant exposure, but the data in their present form, without functional measures, have limitations. It suffices to conclude that nursing infants are exposed to maternal medications. Future avenues to more accurately delineate nursing infant exposure should include preclinical studies of receptor occupancy and of mRNA expression within CNS tissue. Pending the completion of such studies, it is important to provide the data for each individual medication.

Antidepressants in Breast-Feeding: The Data

As a class, antidepressants have been the focus of more published data on breast-feeding than any other class of medications. This database (summarized in Table 5–1) includes 687 separate measures of breast milk concentrations with more than 400 nursing infant serum measures.

The majority of the reports, and of the infant serum measures, involve selective serotonin reuptake inhibitors (SSRIs). There have been numerous attempts to compare the extent of infant exposure and the relative safety of individual antidepressants. A novel approach taken by one group has been the measurement of infant blood serotonin before and during maternal treatment (Epperson et al. 2001, 2003). Although sample sizes are limited,

Table 5–1. Use of antidepressants in breast-feeding women

Medication	Studies	Exposed infants	Infant serum samples	Recommendations			Notes
				PDR	AAP		
SSRIs							
Citalopram[a]	10	69	48	Take into account the risks of citalopram exposure for the infant and the benefits of citalopram treatment for the mother.	Unknown, but may be of concern[†]		Single incident of each of the following reported in exposed infants: colic, decreased feeding, irritability/restlessness, uneasy sleep
Escitalopram	0	0	0	Take into account the risks of escitalopram exposure for the infant and the benefits of escitalopram treatment for the mother.	Unknown, but may be of concern[†]		

Table 5–1. Use of antidepressants in breast-feeding women (*continued*)

Medication	Studies	Exposed infants	Infant serum samples	Recommendations		Notes
				PDR	AAP	
SSRIs (*continued*)						
Fluoxetine[b]	18	202	76	Because fluoxetine is excreted in human milk, nursing while taking fluoxetine is not recommended.	Unknown, but may be of concern	6 nonspecific adverse events reported; 3 infants with colic; 1 had a seizure-like episode; 1 was febrile, somnolent, hypotonic, difficult to arouse; in one study, group of breast-fed infants (*n*=26) overall had less robust weight gain; 1 infant with hyperglycemia and glycosuria; 1 report of unspecified adverse reaction, possibly related to in utero exposure more than to breast milk transfer

Table 5–1. Use of antidepressants in breast-feeding women (*continued*)

Medication	Studies	Exposed infants	Infant serum samples	PDR	AAP	Notes
					Recommendations	
Fluvoxamine[c]	8	16	8	No comment in 2005 PDR	Unknown, but may be of concern	
Paroxetine[d]	13	105	66	Like many other drugs, paroxetine is secreted in human milk, and caution should be exercised when paroxetine is administered to a nursing woman.	Unknown, but may be of concern	1 infant reported to be agitated and unsettled, with difficulty feeding; 1 report of unspecified adverse reaction, possibly related to in utero exposure more than to breast milk transfer

Table 5–1. Use of antidepressants in breast-feeding women *(continued)*

Medication	Studies	Exposed infants	Infant serum samples	Recommendations		Notes
				PDR	AAP	
SSRIs *(continued)*						
Sertraline[e]	18	180	135	It is not known whether sertraline or its metabolites are excreted in human milk, and if so, in what amount. Because many drugs are excreted in human milk, caution should be exercised when sertraline is administered to a nursing woman.	Unknown, but may be of concern	1 report of agitation in an exposed infant; 1 report of somnolence, low muscle tone, hearing problems, and suspected developmental delay in an exposed infant; 7 reports of unspecified adverse reaction possibly related to in utero exposure more than to breast milk transfer
Subtotal		572	333			

Table 5–1. Use of antidepressants in breast-feeding women (*continued*)

Medication	Studies	Exposed infants	Infant serum samples	PDR	Recommendations AAP	Notes
TCAs						
Amitriptyline[f]	2	3	3	No comment in 2005 PDR	Unknown, but may be of concern	
Clomipramine[g]	4	9	9	No comment in 2005 PDR	Unknown, but may be of concern	
Desipramine[h]	1	5	5	Safe use of desipramine during pregnancy and lactation has not been established; therefore, if it is to be given to pregnant patients, nursing mothers, or women of childbearing potential, the possible benefits must be weighed against the possible hazards to mother and child.	Unknown, but may be of concern	

Table 5–1. Use of antidepressants in breast-feeding women (*continued*)

Medication	Studies	Exposed infants	Infant serum samples	PDR	AAP	Notes
					Recommendations	
TCAs (*continued*)						
Dothiepin[i]	3	25	7	Not available in USA	Unknown, but may be of concern	
Doxepin[j]	3	3	3	No comment in 2005 PDR	Unknown, but may be of concern	1 infant reported to have feeding problems, jaundice, hypotonia, vomiting, drowsiness; another with respiratory depression and drowsiness
Imipramine[k]	2	6	6	No comment in 2005 PDR	Unknown, but may be of concern	
Nortriptyline[l]	6	33	33	No comment in 2005 PDR	Unknown, but may be of concern	
Subtotal		84	66			

Table 5–1. Use of antidepressants in breast-feeding women (*continued*)

Medication	Studies	Exposed infants	Infant serum samples	Recommendations		Notes
				PDR	AAP	
Other antidepressants						
Bupropion[m]	4	4	3	Like many other drugs, bupropion and its metabolites are secreted in human milk. Because of the potential for serious adverse reactions in nursing infants from bupropion, a decision should be made whether to discontinue nursing or discontinue the drug, taking into account the importance of the drug to the mother.	Unknown, but may be of concern	Seizure-like episode reported in 1 infant

Table 5–1. Use of antidepressants in breast-feeding women (*continued*)

Medication	Studies	Exposed infants	Infant serum samples	PDR	AAP	Notes
Other antidepressants (*continued*)						
Duloxetine	0	0	0	Duloxetine and/or its metabolites are excreted into the milk of lactating rats. It is unknown whether or not duloxetine and/or its metabolites are excreted into human milk, but nursing while taking duloxetine is not recommended.	Unknown, but may be of concern	
Mirtazapine	0	0	0	No comment in 2005 PDR	Unknown, but may be of concern[†]	
Nefazodone[n]	2	3	0	Not available in USA	Unknown, but may be of concern[†]	1 infant: drowsiness, lethargy, inability to maintain normal body temperature, and feeding problems

	Recommendations	

Table 5-1. Use of antidepressants in breast-feeding women (*continued*)

Medication	Studies	Exposed infants	Infant serum samples	Recommendations		Notes
				PDR	AAP	
Trazodone[o]	1	6	0	No comment in 2005 PDR	Unknown, but may be of concern	
Venlafaxine[p]	5	18	15	Venlafaxine and ODV have been reported to be excreted in human milk. Because of the potential for serious adverse reactions in nursing infants from venlafaxine, a decision should be made whether to discontinue nursing or discontinue the drug, taking into account the importance of the drug to the mother.	Unknown, but may be of concern[†]	
Subtotal		31	18			
Total		687	417			

Table 5–1. Use of antidepressants in breast-feeding women (*continued*)

Medication	Studies	Exposed infants	Infant serum samples	Recommendations		Notes
				PDR	AAP	

Note. AAP=American Academy of Pediatrics; N/A=not mentioned by name or category; ODV=O-desmethylvenlafaxine; PDR=*Physicians' Desk Reference*; SSRI=selective serotonin reuptake inhibitor; TCA=tricyclic antidepressant.

[+]Classified by category (e.g., antidepressants), not by name of drug.

References: [a]Berle et al. 2004; Heikkinen et al. 2002; Hendrick et al. 2003a; Jensen et al. 1997; Lee et al. 2004b; Nordeng et al. 2001; Rampono et al. 2000; Burch and Wells 1992; Schmidt et al. 2000; Spigset et al. 1997; Weissman et al. 2004. [b]Australian Committee 1997, 2003; Berle et al. 2004; Birnbaum et al. 1999; Brent and Wisner 1998; Chambers et al. 1999; Epperson et al. 2003; Hale et al. 2001; Hendrick et al. 2001c 2003___; Isenberg 1990; Kristensen et al. 1999; Lester et al. 1993; Moretti et al. 1999; Suri et al. 2002; Taddio et al. 1996; Weissman et al. 2004; Yoshida et al. 1998a. [c]Arnold et al. 2000; Hagg et al. 2000; Hendrick et al. 2001b, 2003a ; Kristensen et al. 2002; Nordeng et al. 2001; Piontek et al. 2001; Weissman et al. 2004; Yoshida et al. 1997b. [d]Australian Committee 1997, 2003; Begg et al. 1999; Berle et al. 2004; Birnbaum et al. 1999; Hendrick et al. 2000, 2001a, 2003a; Misri et al. 2000; Nordeng et al. 2001; Ohman et al. 1999; Stowe et al. 2000; Weissman et al. 2004. [e]Altshuler et al. 1995; Australian Committee 1997, 2003; Berle et al. 2004; Birnbaum et al. 1999; Dodd et al. 2000b, 2001; Epperson et al. 1997, 2001; Hendrick et al. 2001b, 2003a; Kristensen et al. 1998; Mammen et al. 1997; Stowe et al. 1997, 2003; Weissman et al. 2004; Wisner et al. 1998. [f]Breyer-Pfaff et al. 1995; Yoshida et al. 1997a. [g]Birnbaum et al. 1999; Schimmell et al. 1991; Wisner et al. 1995; Yoshida et al. 1997a. [h]Birnbaum et al. 1999. [i]Ilett et al. 1992; Buist and Janson 1995; Yoshida et al. 1997a. [j]Frey et al. 1999; Kemp et al. 1985; Matheson et al. 1985. [k]Birnbaum et al. 1999; Yoshida et al. 1997a. [l]Altshuler et al. 1995; Birnbaum et al. 1999; Weissman et al. 2004; Wisner and Perel 1991, 1996; Wisner et al. 1997. [m]Baab et al. 2002; Briggs et al. 1993; Chaudron and Schoenecker 2004; Haas et al. 2004. [n]Dodd et al. 2000a; Yapp et al. 2000. [o]Verbeeck et al. 1986. [p]Berle et al. 2004; Hendrick et al. 2001a, 2003a; Ilett et al. 1998, 2002.

no significant change in plasma serotonin was demonstrated during fluoxetine ($n=11$) or sertraline ($n=14$) therapy.

It is noteworthy that the lactation categories for SSRI antidepressants listed in the PDR and AAP guidelines (i.e., "unknown, but may be of concern") do not reflect the extant literature. The best example of the limitation of the PDR in this area is the statement regarding sertraline ("it is not known whether and if so to what amount sertraline and its metabolites are excreted into human milk")—a medication with the greatest amount of data on breast milk excretion of any medication in the PDR. Antidepressant use during lactation warrants continued concern; however, the failure of the AAP to cite the extant data set in its latest report is inexplicable. A literature review identified 11 publications, comprising 40 infants (5.2% of total published breast-feeding cases), that noted purportedly adverse effects on the infant from antidepressant exposure during breast-feeding. An empirically conservative appraisal of these reports is warranted, given the ready availability of alternative feeding methods. In the absence of controlled studies, the greatest evidence for causality that can be derived from the available case literature is that in some instances the infant symptoms resolved when breast-feeding was discontinued. In any event, the preponderance of adverse events consists of colic, other gastrointestinal disturbances, and sleep disruptions. To put it simply, the clinician, patient, and family must weigh the potential for antidepressant-associated gastrointestinal distress and difficulty sleeping in the infant versus the benefits of breast-feeding. The principal exception to this rule is doxepin, which in two cases appeared to cause clinically significant adverse effects in a nursing infant.

Antidepressants in Breast-Feeding: Infant Monitoring

Routine breast milk and/or nursing infant serum sampling is not indicated by the current literature. The accuracy of such measures outside of a research laboratory would be suspect, and the antidepressants are not associated with alterations in other laboratory indices—with limited exceptions such as the syndrome of inappropriate antidiuretic hormone. It is important to note that data on the placental passage of antidepressants (Hendrick et al. 2003b; Z.N. Stowe, unpublished data) have demonstrated umbilical cord concentrations at delivery ranging from 40% to over 100% of maternal serum concentrations. By comparison, a nursing infant would have to breast-feed exclusively for more than 2 years to accrue the level of antidepressant exposure that occurs during a single month of pregnancy. Furthermore, newborn infants have a full complement of metabolic enzymes and α_1-glycoprotein concentrations, comparable to those of adults. Therefore, concern about antidepressant exposure via breast milk, in cases where exposure during pregnancy has already occurred, is overstated.

Mood Stabilizers in Breast-Feeding: The Data

The pharmacologic armamentarium for the treatment of bipolar disorder continues to expand. A variety of medications—antiepileptic medications, lithium carbonate, and antipsychotic medications—are used in the treatment of bipolar disorder. The literature on their use during breast-feeding is summarized in Table 5–2.

The bulk of the breast milk data on anticonvulsants is derived from women with epilepsy and includes 23 separate reports. Remarkably, nursing infant serum has been measured in only 59 infants. In contrast to the PDR, the AAP considers carbamazepine and valproate to be potentially compatible with breast-feeding. It is difficult to discern the meaning of *compatible* or exactly which variables (total number of individual cases, estimates of nursing infant dose) drive the categorization. The "compatible" rating is particularly surprising given that the purported adverse effects are consistent with the potentially hazardous side effects of these medications.

Lamotrigine has garnered increased attention in the treatment of bipolar disorder and is a unique medication with respect to breast-feeding. Because it is exclusively metabolized via glucuronidation, a metabolic pathway that is immature in the neonate, concerns have been raised with respect to lamotrigine and breast-feeding. No adverse effects have been documented among infants exposed to lamotrigine during nursing, with M/P ratios collectively equaling about 0.6 (Liporace et al. 2004; Ohman et al. 2000; Rambeck et al. 1997; Tomson et al. 1997). The small case series by

Table 5–2. Use of mood stabilizers/antiepileptic medications in breast-feeding women

Medication	Studies	Exposed infants	Infant serum samples	Recommendations		Notes
				PDR	AAP	
Anticonvulsants						
Carbamazepine[a]	11	51	10	Carbamazepine and its epoxide metabolite are transferred to breast milk. Because of the potential for serious adverse reactions in nursing infants from carbamazepine, a decision should be made whether to discontinue nursing or to discontinue the drug in nursing women, taking into account the importance of the drug to the mother.	Usually compatible with breast-feeding	2 cases of cholestatic hepatitis, 1 case of elevated GGT, 1 "seizure-like" episode, 2 "hyperexcitable" infants
Lamotrigine[b]	4	16	16	Preliminary data indicate that lamotrigine passes into human milk. Because the effects on the infant exposed to lamotrigine by this route are unknown, breast-feeding while taking lamotrigine is not recommended.	Unknown, but may be of concern	Infant concentrations up to 30% of maternal concentrations

Table 5–2. Use of mood stabilizers/antiepileptic medications in breast-feeding women (*continued*)

Medication	Studies	Exposed infants	Infant serum samples	PDR	Recommendations		Notes
					AAP		
Anticonvulsants (*continued*)							
Levetiracetam[c]	1	0	0	Levetiracetam is excreted in breast milk. Because of the potential for serious adverse reactions in nursing infants from levetiracetam, a decision should be made whether to discontinue nursing or discontinue the drug in nursing women, taking into account the importance of the drug to the mother.	N/A		High concentration in breast milk
Oxcarbazepine[d]	2	2	1	Oxcarbazepine is excreted in breast milk. Because of the potential for serious adverse reactions in nursing infants from oxcarbazepine, a decision should be made whether to discontinue nursing or discontinue the drug in nursing women, taking into account the importance of the drug to the mother.	N/A		

Table 5–2. Use of mood stabilizers/antiepileptic medications in breast-feeding women (*continued*)

Medication	Studies	Exposed infants	Infant serum samples	Recommendations		Notes
				PDR	AAP	
Topiramate[e]	1	3	3	Topiramate is excreted in the milk of lactating rats. The excretion of topiramate in human milk has not been evaluated in controlled studies. Limited observations in patients suggest an extensive secretion of topiramate into breast milk. Since many drugs are excreted in human milk, and because the potential for serious adverse reactions in nursing infants to topiramate is unknown, the potential benefit to mother should be weighed against the potential risk to the infant when considering recommendations regarding nursing.	N/A	

Table 5–2. Use of mood stabilizers/antiepileptic medications in breast-feeding women *(continued)*

| Medication | Studies | Exposed infants | Infant serum samples | Recommendations | | Notes |
				PDR	AAP	
Anticonvulsants *(continued)*						
Valproic acid[f]	10	38	27	Valproic acid is excreted in breast milk. It is not known what effect this has on a nursing infant. Consideration should be given to discontinuing nursing when valproic acid is administered to a breast-feeding woman.	Usually compatible with breast-feeding	1 infant with thrombocytopenia and anemia
Subtotal	110	57				

Table 5–2. Use of mood stabilizers/antiepileptic medications in breast-feeding women (continued)

Medication	Studies	Exposed infants	Infant serum samples	PDR	Recommendations AAP	Notes
Atypical antipsychotics						
Aripiprazole	0	0	0	It is not known whether aripiprazole or its metabolites are excreted in human milk. It is recommended that women receiving aripiprazole not breast-feed.	Unknown, but may be of concern[†]	
Clozapine[g]	1	0	0	Animal studies suggest that clozapine may be excreted in breast milk and have an effect on the nursing infant. Therefore, women receiving clozapine should not breast-feed.	Unknown, but may be of concern	
Olanzapine[h]	6	16	7	It is not known if olanzapine is excreted in human milk. It is recommended that women receiving olanzapine not breast-feed.	Unknown, but may be of concern[†]	

Use of Antidepressants and Mood Stabilizers in Breast-Feeding Women 125

Table 5–2. Use of mood stabilizers/antiepileptic medications in breast-feeding women (*continued*)

Medication	Studies	Exposed infants	Infant serum samples	PDR	Recommendations AAP	Notes
Atypical antipsychotics (*continued*)						
Quetiapine[j]	1	1	0	It is not known if quetiapine is excreted in human milk. It is recommended that women receiving quetiapine not breast-feed.	Unknown, but may be of concern[†]	
Risperidone[j]	3	4	2	Risperidone and 9-hydroxyris-peridone are excreted in human breast milk. Therefore, women receiving risperidone should not breast-feed.	Unknown, but may be of concern[†]	
Ziprasidone	0	0	0	It is not known whether, and in what amount, ziprasidone or its metabolites are excreted in human milk. It is recommended that women receiving ziprasidone not breast-feed.	Unknown, but may be of concern[†]	
Subtotal	21		9			

Table 5–2. Use of mood stabilizers/antiepileptic medications in breast-feeding women (*continued*)

Medication	Studies	Exposed infants	Infant serum samples	PDR	AAP	Notes
Lithium[k]	8	22	12	Lithium is excreted in human milk. Nursing should not be undertaken during lithium therapy except in rare and unusual circumstances where, in the view of the physician, the potential benefits to the mother outweigh possible hazards to the child.	Should be given to nursing mothers with caution	1 case of lithium toxicity with infant concentration at 1.4 mEq/L; 1 infant with cyanosis and lethargy; ECG changes in 3 infants
Subtotal		22	12			
Total		153	78			

Table 5–2. Use of mood stabilizers/antiepileptic medications in breast-feeding women (*continued*)

Medication	Studies	Exposed infants	Infant serum samples	Recommendations		
				PDR	AAP	Notes

Note. AAP=American Academy of Pediatrics; ECG=electrocardiographic; GGT=γ-glutamyltransaminase; N/A=not mentioned by name or category; PDR=*Physicians' Desk Reference.*

†Classified by category (e.g., antipsychotics), not by name of drug.

References: [a]Brent and Wisner 1998; Frey et al. 1990, 2002; Froescher et al. 1984; Kaneko et al. 1979; Kok et al. 1982; Kuhnz et al. 1983; Merlob et al. 1992; Niebyl et al. 1979; Pynnonen and Sillanpaa 1975; Pynnonen et al. 1977; Wisner and Perel 1998.

[b]Liporace et al. 2004; Ohman et al. 2000; Rambeck et al. 1997; Tomson et al. 1997.

[c]Kramer et al. 2002.

[d]Bulau et al. 1988; Gentile 2003.

[e]Ohman et al. 2002.

[f]Alexander 1979; Birnbaum et al. 1999; Dickinson et al. 1979; Nau et al. 1981; Philbert et al. 1985; Piontek et al. 2000; Stahl et al. 1997; Tsuru et al. 1988; von Unruh et al. 1984; Wisner and Perel 1998.

[g]Barnas et al. 1994.

[h]Ambresin et al. 2004; Croke et al. 2002; Friedman et al. 2003; Gardiner et al. 2003; Goldstein et al. 2000; Kirchheiner et al. 2000; Lee et al. 2004a.

[i]Hill et al. 2000; Ilett et al. 2004; Ratnayake and Libretto 2002.

[k]Fries 1970; Moretti et al. 2003; Schou and Amdisen 1973; Skausig and Schou 1977; Sykes et al. 1976; Tunnessen and Hertz 1972; Weinstein and Goldfield 1969; Woody et al. 1971.

Ohman et al. (2000) indicated that serum concentrations of lamotrigine in nursing infants are approximately 30% of maternal concentrations. No incidence of rash has been reported.

The use of lithium in lactating women has been contraindicated historically. Adverse events, including lethargy, hypotonia, hypothermia, cyanosis, and electrocardiographic changes, were reported in three children (Skausig and Schou 1977; Tunnessen and Hertz 1972; Woody et al. 1971), including one infant who developed frank lithium toxicity with a serum concentration of 1.4 mEq/L, which was double the maternal serum concentration (Skausig and Schou 1977). The AAP consequently discourages the use of lithium during lactation (American Academy of Pediatrics 2001). Because dehydration and nonsteroidal anti-inflammatory drugs (NSAIDs) may increase the risk for elevated lithium levels, the hydration status of nursing infants of mothers taking lithium should be carefully monitored, and these children should not be administered ibuprofen or other NSAIDs.

The atypical antipsychotics currently available in the United States include aripiprazole, clozapine, olanzapine, quetiapine, risperidone, and ziprasidone. These medications are now first-line agents for psychotic disorders, and most are approved for the management of acute mania. The use of these agents has also expanded to other disorders, including obsessive-compulsive disorder and refractory depression. Despite increased utilization, there are sparse data on use of these drugs in lactating women, with fewer than a dozen cases reported. As with other classes of psychotropic medications, these limited studies demonstrate that these medications are present in human breast milk.

The only investigation of the perinatal pharmacokinetics (PK) of clozapine demonstrated similar medication concentrations in maternal serum and amniotic fluid but markedly higher concentrations in fetal serum and breast milk (Barnas et al. 1994), leading the authors to conclude that clozapine accumulates in the fetal circulation and in breast milk. Although no cases of agranulocytosis have been reported in the infants of women taking clozapine during lactation, this theoretical risk and the consequent requirement for monitoring of leukocyte counts in nursing infants limit the utility of clozapine.

Case reports of 16 infants exposed to olanzapine during lactation with no evidence of infant toxicity currently appear in the literature (Croke et al. 2002; Friedman and Rosenthal 2003; Gardiner et al. 2003; Goldstein et al. 2000; Kirchheiner et al. 2000). PK studies of olanzapine during lactation reported that no plasma concentrations were detectable during nursing in 6 infants (Gardiner et al. 2003; Kirchheiner et al. 2000) and that the median infant daily dose via breast-feeding was approximately 1.0%–1.6% of the maternal dose (Ambresin et al. 2004; Croke et al. 2002; Gardiner et al. 2003).

The reproductive safety literature for risperidone is limited to case reports of four women who were administered risperidone during gestation and while nursing, with no evidence of complications in nursing infants (Ilett et al. 2004; Ratnayake and Libretto 2002). PK studies of risperidone excretion into breast milk reported M/P ratios of less than 0.5 for both risperidone and 9-hydroxyrisperidone (Hill et al. 2000; Ilett et al. 2004) and infant doses ranging from 2.3% to 4.7% of the maternal dose (Ilett et al. 2004). A single case of quetiapine use during lactation following use during pregnancy estimated the nursing infant dose at 0.09% of the maternal daily dose (Lee et al. 2004a). There are currently no reports regarding the use of aripiprazole or ziprasidone during lactation.

Despite the use of typical antipsychotic medications for more than four decades, there are limited case reports for use during lactation. PK studies of haloperidol (Stewart et al. 1980; Whalley et al. 1981; Yoshida et al. 1998b), trifluoperazine (Wilson et al. 1980; Yoshida et al. 1998b), perphenazine (Wilson et al. 1980), thioxanthenes (Matheson and Skjaeraasen 1988), and chlorpromazine (Yoshida et al. 1998b) have uniformly reported an M/P ratio of less than 1.0. Nursing infant serum measures have not been reported.

In summary, the anticonvulsants account for the majority of data in lactating women for the mood-stabilizing medications. The limited nature of the data on use of antipsychotics, both atypical and typical, precludes any meaningful summary.

Mood Stabilizers in Breast-Feeding: Infant Monitoring

In contrast to antidepressants, mood stabilizers might directly affect laboratory indices in the breast-feeding infant. There is no consensus with respect to infant monitoring, although a conservative approach warrants monitoring of those indices that are potentially affected by the individual medications. It would be prudent to establish a baseline and to periodically repeat such measures. Like the antidepressants, all mood stabilizers studied to date cross the placental barrier. Typically, anticonvulsant and lithium exposure in pregnancy is greater than 80% and breast-feeding exposure is considerably less.

In summary, the literature on antidepressants and mood stabilizers has grown considerably in recent years. There is no evidence that antidepressants pose an acute risk to nursing infants. The mood stabilizers present a more complex issue with respect to both acute safety and the need for infant monitoring. Pending the completion of long-term follow-up studies specifically targeting exposure via breast milk, the issue will remain relative safety. These data must be viewed in the context of the potential risk that untreated maternal mood disorders may pose to infant well-being.

Mental Illness in Postpartum Women: Spectrum of Psychiatric Conditions

The treatment of mental illness during lactation represents a complicated clinical situation that involves the health and well-being of at least two individuals, the mother and the child. The question regarding use of medications during lactation is one of "relative safety" that must consider both the safety of available therapies and the impact of maternal illness. Numerous laboratory and clinical investigations have demonstrated that maternal depression, anxiety, and stress can produce a wide spectrum of adverse effects on the offspring.

Briefly, the literature includes more than 20,000 mother-infant pairs (Ragan et al. 2003) in a variety of study designs demonstrating deleterious consequences for the children of women with depression. For example, infants of depressed mothers exhibit aberrant behavior, including decreased facial expression, less head orientation, less crying, and increased fussiness, as early as age 3 months (Martinez et al. 1996). Older children of depressed mothers display ineffective emotional regulation (Downey and

Coyne 1990), delayed motor development (Galler et al. 2000), poor interpersonal interactions (Jameson et al. 1997), lower self-esteem (Downey and Coyne 1990), more fear and anxiety (Lyons-Ruth et al. 2000), greater aggression (Jameson et al. 1997), and insecure and disorganized attachment behaviors (Martins and Gaffan 2000). Long-term investigations have demonstrated increased emotional instability, suicidal behavior, and behavioral problems in children of depressed mothers, and these children are more likely to require psychiatric treatment (Lyons-Ruth et al. 2000; Weissman et al. 1984). Consistent with this pattern, two recent studies found that maternal depression in the first postnatal year was associated with elevated cortisol and attention deficits (Essex et al. 2002) and predicted increased violent behavior in 10- to 13-year-olds (Maki et al. 2003).

Data regarding the effect of other maternal mood disorders, such as bipolar disorder, are limited. In contrast, a recent prospective investigation demonstrated that prenatal maternal anxiety, a known risk factor for depression in the postpartum period, is related to anxiety and attention-deficit/hyperactivity disorder symptoms in school-age children (Van den Bergh and Marcoen 2004). These clinical data are complemented by an extensive animal literature in a variety of species demonstrating that stress during the early postpartum period adversely affects offspring growth, learning ability, and postnatal development, giving rise to varied biobehavioral aberrations that persist into adulthood (for a review, see Newport et al. 2002).

In summary, the potential effects of untreated maternal psychopathology are potentially more devastating than the effects of other medical conditions routinely treated in lactating women.

Clinical Decision Making

The clinician is reminded that breast-feeding is a recommendation, not a mandate. The option of weaning should always be considered. However, the emphasis on the importance of breast milk has fostered a doctrinaire commitment on the part of many women to breast-feed. Similarly, the PDR and the AAP have obviously taken a very conservative approach, making blanket categorizations that often do not reflect the current literature and as such are of limited utility in treatment planning. Instead, the discrepancy between the published data and these guidelines establishes an arena of discrepant opinions that potentially invites increased medicolegal liability and increased clinician and patient anxiety. An ethical question warrants consideration: Should the infants of women with mental illness and the women themselves be deprived of the potential benefits of breast-feeding secondary to their mental illness?

Our group has proposed and continues to refine a model aimed at minimizing infant exposure, as a guide to clinical decision making during the postpartum (Newport et al. 2001; Stowe et al. 2001). For example, if a breast-feeding mother is more likely to consume alcohol, smoke cigarettes, or take other medications (both prescription and over-the-counter) when she is depressed or anxious, these alternative exposures should be considered in the treatment planning. When treatment is indicated, the options for breast-feeding women are reasonably straightforward: 1) use nonpharmacologic treatments, 2) wean and initiate pharmacologic treatment, and 3) continue to breast-feed and initiate pharmacologic treatment. Neither nontreatment nor delayed treatment is a reasonable option. Additional steps to minimize risk for the third option include the following:

1. Use a medication appropriate for the diagnosis and for any comorbid conditions.
2. Use a medication to which the patient has had a prior response. The postpartum breast-feeding patient should not experiment with new medications.
3. Use a medication to which the infant has had prior exposure. If a patient has taken a particular medication during pregnancy (even if it was discontinued at knowledge of conception), and it was clinically effective, then the choice for breast-feeding has already been made. Switching medications is not recommended (Med A in pregnancy+Med B in lactation=no/limited data).
4. Use a medication for which there are published data ("new and improved"=no/limited data).

---

5. Monotherapy at any dose is preferable to introducing a second medication in women who are breast-feeding.
6. Infant serum monitoring is not recommended in the clinical setting for antidepressants. If adverse effects are suspected, suspend breast-feeding.
7. Infant serum monitoring for mood stabilizers should reflect the indices affected by the individual medications. These measures should include a baseline measure, with repeated measures once maternal steady state is attained. If adverse effects are suspected or if a change in infant laboratory indices is observed, breast-feeding should be suspended pending additional follow-up and discussion with the patient.
8. If unsure, get a consultation. There are several Web sites devoted to women's mental health and the reproductive safety of psychotropic medications. Many of these links are available through http://www.emorywomensprogram.org.

Conclusion

Psychiatric treatment of breast-feeding women will remain a fertile ground for scientific investigation and vigorous debate. A woman's desire to breast-feed may complicate psychiatric treatment, but it by no means precludes it. Given the multidisciplinary professional support for breast-feeding, we are responsible for advancing our knowledge of appropriate treatments and for establishing monitoring guidelines. This responsibility mandates extending the data on the impact of maternal mood disorders on the constituents of breast milk and understanding the impact on successful breast-feeding. Additional detailed pharmacokinetic investigations will enhance our understanding of nursing infant exposure and the role of pharmacogenomics in determining infant exposures.

Psychiatry, as a subspecialty, has accumulated considerable data regarding psychotropic medications in lactation. It remains worrisome that other specialties lag behind in the collection of data, yet continue to expand the stigma associated with mental illness by rendering potentially erroneous conclusions and failing to note the extant literature.

References

Alexander FW: Sodium valproate and pregnancy (letter). Arch Dis Child 54:240, 1979

Altshuler LL, Burt VK, McMullen M, et al: Breast-feeding and sertraline: a 24-hour analysis. J Clin Psychiatry 56:243–245, 1995

Ambresin G, Berney P, Schulz P, et al: Olanzapine excretion into breast milk: a case report. J Clin Psychopharmacol 24:93–95, 2004

American Academy of Pediatrics, Committee on Drugs: Transfer of drugs and other chemicals into human milk. Pediatrics 108:776–789, 2001

Arnold L, Suckow RF, Lichtenstein PK: Fluvoxamine concentrations in breast milk and maternal and infant sera. J Clin Psychopharmacol 20:491–493, 2000

Australian Adverse Drug Reactions Advisory Committee: SSRIs and neonatal disorders: breast milk transfer. Australian Adverse Drug Reactions Bulletin 16(4), 1997

Australian Adverse Drug Reactions Advisory Committee: Maternal SSRI use and neonatal effects. Australian Adverse Drug Reactions Bulletin 22(4):14, 2003

Baab SW, Peindl KS, Piontek CM, et al: Serum bupropion levels in 2 breastfeeding mother-infant pairs. J Clin Psychiatry 63:910–911, 2002

Barnas C, Bergant A, Hummer M, et al: Clozapine concentrations in maternal and fetal plasma, amniotic fluid, and breast milk (letter). Am J Psychiatry 151:945, 1994

Begg EJ, Duffull SB, Saunders DA, et al: Paroxetine in human milk. Br J Clin Pharmacol 48:142–147, 1999

Berle JO, Steen VM, Aamo TO, et al: Breastfeeding during maternal antidepressant treatment with serotonin reuptake inhibitors: infant exposure, clinical symptoms, and cytochrome P450 genotypes. J Clin Psychiatry 65:1228–1234, 2004

Birnbaum CS, Cohen LS, Bailey JW, et al: Serum concentrations of antidepressants and benzodiazepines in nursing infants: a case series. Pediatrics 104:e11, 1999

Brent NB, Wisner KL: Fluoxetine and carbamazepine concentrations in a nursing mother/infant pair. Clin Pediatr (Phila) 37:41–44, 1998

Breyer-Pfaff U, Nill K, Entenmann KN, et al: Secretion of amitriptyline and metabolites into breast milk (letter). Am J Psychiatry 152:812–813, 1995

Briggs GG, Samson JH, Ambrose PJ, et al: Excretion of bupropion in breast milk. Ann Pharmacother 27:431–433, 1993

Buist A, Janson H: Effect of exposure to dothiepin and northiaden in breast milk on child development. Br J Psychiatry 167:370–373, 1995

Bulau P, Paar WD, von Unruh GE: Pharmacokinetics of oxcarbazepine and 10-hydroxy-carbazepine in the newborn child of an oxcarbazepine-treated mother. Eur J Clin Pharmacol 34:311–313, 1988

Burch KJ, Wells BG: Fluoxetine/norfluoxetine concentrations in human milk. Pediatrics 89:676–677, 1992

Chambers CD, Anderson PO, Thomas RG, et al: Weight gain in infants breastfed by mothers who take fluoxetine. Pediatrics 104(5):e61, 1999

Chaudron LH, Schoenecker CJ: Bupropion and breastfeeding: a case of a possible infant seizure. J Clin Psychiatry 65:881–882, 2004

Cohen LS, Nonacs R, Viguera AC, et al: Diagnosis and treatment of depression during pregnancy. CNS Spectr 9:209–216, 2004

Croke S, Buist A, Hackett LP, et al: Olanzapine excretion in human breast milk: estimation of infant exposure. Int J Neuropsychopharmacol 5:243–247, 2002

Dickinson RG, Harland RC, Lynn RK, et al: Transmission of valproic acid (Depakene) across the placenta: half-life of the drug in mother and baby. J Pediatr 94:832–835, 1979

Dodd S, Maguire KP, Burrows GD, et al: Nefazodone in the breast milk of nursing mothers: a report of two patients. J Clin Psychopharmacol 20:717–718, 2000a

Dodd S, Stocky A, Buist A, et al: Sertraline in paired blood plasma and breast-milk samples from nursing mothers. Hum Psychopharmacol 15:261–264, 2000b

Dodd S, Stocky A, Buist A, et al: Sertraline analysis in the plasma of breast-fed infants. Aust NZ J Psychiatry 35:545–546, 2001

Downey G, Coyne JC: Children of depressed parents: an integrative review. Psychol Bull 108:50–76, 1990

Epperson CN, Anderson GM, McDougle CJ: Sertraline and breast-feeding. N Engl J Med 336:1189–1190, 1997

Epperson CN, Czarkowski KA, Ward-O'Brien D, et al: Maternal sertraline treatment and serotonin transport in breast-feeding mother-infant pairs. Am J Psychiatry 158:1631–1637, 2001

Epperson CN, Jatlow PI, Czarkowski K, et al: Maternal fluoxetine treatment in the postpartum period: effects on platelet serotonin and plasma drug levels in breastfeeding mother-infant pairs. Pediatrics 112(5):e425–e429, 2003

Essex MJ, Klein MH, Cho E, et al: Maternal stress beginning in infancy may sensitize children to later stress exposure: effects on cortisol and behavior. Biol Psychiatry 52:776–784, 2002

Frey B, Schubiger G, Musy JP: Transient cholestatic hepatitis in a neonate associated with carbamazepine exposure during pregnancy and breast-feeding. Eur J Pediatr 150:136–138, 1990

Frey B, Braegger CP, Ghelfi D: Neonatal cholestatic hepatitis from carbamazepine exposure during pregnancy and breast feeding. Ann Pharmacother 36:644–647, 2002

Frey OR, Scheidt P, von Brenndorff AI: Adverse effects in a newborn infant breast-fed by a mother treated with doxepin. Ann Pharmacother 33:690–693, 1999

Friedman SH, Rosenthal MB: Treatment of perinatal delusional disorder: a case report. Int J Psychiatry Med 33:391–394, 2003

Fries H: Lithium in pregnancy. Lancet 1(7658):1233, 1970

Froescher W, Eichelbaum M, Niesen M, et al: Carbamazepine levels in breast milk. Ther Drug Monit 6:266–271, 1984

Galler JR, Harrison RH, Ramsey F, et al: Maternal depressive symptoms affect infant cognitive development in Barbados. J Child Psychol Psychiatry 41:747–757, 2000

Gardiner SJ, Kristensen JH, Begg EJ, et al: Transfer of olanzapine into breast milk, calculation of infant drug dose, and effect on breast-fed infants. Am J Psychiatry 160:1428–1431, 2003

Gentile S: Oxcarbazepine in pregnancy and lactation (letter). Clin Drug Invest 23:687, 2003

Goldstein DJ, Corbin LA, Fung MC: Olanzapine-exposed pregnancies and lactation: early experience. J Clin Psychopharmacol 20:399–403, 2000

Haas JS, Kaplan CP, Barenboim D, et al: Bupropion in breast milk: an exposure assessment for potential treatment to prevent post-partum tobacco use. Tob Control 13:52–56, 2004

Hagg S, Granberg K, Carleborg L: Excretion of fluvoxamine into breast milk. Br J Clin Pharmacol 49:286–288, 2000

Hale TW, Shum S, Grossberg M: Fluoxetine toxicity in a breastfed infant. Clin Pediatr 40:681–684, 2001

Heikkinen T, Ekblad U, Kero P, et al: Citalopram in pregnancy and lactation. Clin Pharmacol Ther 72:184–191, 2002

Hendrick V, Altshuler L: Management of major depression during pregnancy. Am J Psychiatry 159:1667–1673, 2002

Hendrick V, Stowe ZN, Altshuler LL, et al: Paroxetine use during breast-feeding. J Clin Psychopharmacol 20:587–589, 2000

Hendrick V, Altshuler L, Wertheimer A, et al: Venlafaxine and breast-feeding (letter). Am J Psychiatry 158:2089–2090, 2001a

Hendrick V, Fukuchi A, Altshuler L, et al: Use of sertraline, paroxetine, and fluvoxamine in nursing women. Br J Psychiatry 179:163–166, 2001b

Hendrick V, Stowe ZN, Altshuler LL, et al: Fluoxetine and norfluoxetine concentrations in nursing infants and breast milk. Biol Psychiatry 50: 775–782, 2001c

Hendrick V, Smith LM, Hwang S, et al: Weight gain in breastfed infants of mothers taking antidepressant medications. J Clin Psychiatry 64:410–412, 2003a

Hendrick V, Stowe Z, Altshuler LL, et al: Placental passage of anti-depressant medications. Am J Psychiatry 160:993–996, 2003b

Hill RC, McIvor RJ, Wojnar-Horton RE, et al: Risperidone distribution and excretion into human milk: case report and estimated infant exposure during breast-feeding. J Clin Psychopharmacol 20:285–286, 2000

Ilett KF, Lebedevs TH, Wojnar-Horton RE, et al: The excretion of dothie-pin and its primary metabolites in breast milk. Br J Clin Pharmacol 33:635–639, 1992

Ilett KF, Hackett LP, Dusci LJ, et al: Distribution and excretion of ven-lafaxine and O-desmethylvenlafaxine in human milk. Br J Clin Pharmacol 45:459–462, 1998

Ilett KF, Kristensen JH, Hackett LP, et al: Distribution of venlafaxine and its O-desmethyl metabolite in human milk and their effects in breast-fed infants. Br J Clin Pharmacol 53:17–22, 2002

Ilett KF, Hackett LP, Kristensen JH, et al: Transfer of risperidone and 9-hydroxyrisperidone into human milk. Ann Pharmacother 38:273–276, 2004

Isenberg KE: Excretion of fluoxetine in human breast milk (letter). J Clin Psychiatry 51(4):169, 1990

Jameson PB, Gelfand DM, Kulcsar E, et al: Mother-toddler interaction patterns associated with maternal depression. Dev Psychopathol 9:537–550, 1997

Jensen PN, Olesen OV, Bertelsen A, et al: Citalopram and desmethyl-citalopram concentrations in breast milk and in serum of mother and infant. Ther Drug Monit 19:236–239, 1997

Kaneko S, Sato T, Suzuki K: The levels of anticonvulsants in breast milk. Br J Clin Pharmacol 7:624–627, 1979

Kemp J, Ilett KF, Booth J, et al: Excretion of doxepin and N-desmethyl-doxepin in human milk. Br J Clin Pharmacol 20:497–499, 1985

Kirchheiner J, Berghofer A, Bolk-Weischedel D: Healthy outcome under olanzapine treatment in a pregnant woman. Pharmacopsychiatry 33: 78–80, 2000

Kok TH, Taitz LS, Bennett MJ, et al: Drowsiness due to clemastine trans-mitted in breast milk. Lancet 1(8277):914–915, 1982

Kramer G, Hosli I, Glanzmann R, et al: Levetiracetam accumulation in human breast milk (abstract). Epilepsia 43 (suppl 7):105, 2002

Kristensen JH, Ilett KF, Dusci LJ, et al: Distribution and excretion of sertraline and N-desmethylsertraline in human milk. Br J Clin Pharmacol 45:453–457, 1998

Kristensen JH, Ilett KF, Hackett LP, et al: Distribution and excretion of fluoxetine and norfluoxetine in human milk. Br J Clin Pharmacol 48:521–527, 1999

Kristensen JH, Hackett LP, Kohan R, et al: The amount of fluvoxamine in milk is unlikely to be a cause of adverse effects in breastfed infants. J Hum Lact 18:139–143, 2002

Kuhnz W, Jager-Roman E, Rating D, et al: Carbamazepine and carbamazepine-10,11-epoxide during pregnancy and postnatal period in epileptic mothers and their nursed infants: pharmacokinetics and clinical effects. Pediatr Pharmacol (New York) 3:199–208, 1983

Lee A, Giesbrecht E, Dunn E, et al: Excretion of quetiapine in breast milk. Am J Psychiatry 161:1715–1716, 2004a

Lee A, Woo J, Ito S: Frequency of infant adverse events that are associated with citalopram use during pregnancy. Am J Obstet Gynecol 190:218–221, 2004b

Lester BM, Cucca J, Andreozzi L, et al: Possible association between fluoxetine hydrochloride and colic in an infant. J Am Acad Child Adolesc Psychiatry 32:1253–1255, 1993

Liporace J, Kao A, D'Abreu A: Concerns regarding lamotrigine and breast-feeding. Epilepsy Behav 5:102–105, 2004

Lyons-Ruth K, Wolfe R, Lyubchik A: Depression and the parenting of young children: making the case for early preventive mental health services. Harv Rev Psychiatry 8:148–153, 2000

Maki P, Veijola J, Rasanen P, et al: Criminality in the offspring of antenatally depressed mothers: a 33-year follow-up of the Northern Finland 1966 Birth Cohort. J Affect Disord 74:273–278, 2003

Mammen OK, Perel JM, Rudolph G, et al: Sertraline and norsertraline levels in three breastfed infants. J Clin Psychiatry 58:100–103, 1997

Martinez A, Malphurs J, Field T, et al: Depressed mothers' and their infants' interactions with nondepressed partners. Infant Mental Health Journal 17:74–80, 1996

Martins C, Gaffan EA: Effects of early maternal depression on patterns of infant-mother attachment: a meta-analytic investigation. J Child Psychol Psychiatry 41:737–746, 2000

Matheson I, Skjaeraasen J: Milk concentrations of flupenthixol, nortriptyline and zuclopenthixol and between-breast differences in two patients. Eur J Clin Pharmacol 35:217–220, 1988

Matheson I, Pande H, Alertsen AR: Respiratory depression caused by N-desmethyldoxepin in breast milk. Lancet 2(8464):1124, 1985

Merlob P, Mor N, Litwin A: Transient hepatic dysfunction in an infant of an epileptic mother treated with carbamazepine during pregnancy and lactation. Ann Pharmacother 26:1563–1565, 1992

Misri S, Kim J, Riggs KW, et al: Paroxetine levels in postpartum depressed women, breast milk, and infant serum. J Clin Psychiatry 61:828–832, 2000

Moretti ME, Sharma A, Bar-Oz B, et al: Fluoxetine and its effects on the nursing infant: a prospective cohort study (abstract). Clin Pharmacol Ther 65:141, 1999

Moretti ME, Koren G, Verjee Z, et al: Monitoring lithium in breast milk: an individualized approach for breast-feeding mothers. Ther Drug Monit 25:364–366, 2003

Nau H, Rating D, Koch S, et al: Valproic acid and its metabolites: placental transfer, neonatal pharmacokinetics, transfer via mother's milk and clinical status in neonates of epileptic mothers. J Pharmacol Exp Ther 219:768–777, 1981

Newport DJ, Stowe ZN: Clinical management of perinatal depression: focus on paroxetine. Psychopharmacol Bull 37 (suppl 1):148–166, 2003

Newport DJ, Wilcox MM, Stowe ZN: Antidepressants during pregnancy and lactation: defining exposure and treatment issues. Semin Perinatol 25:177–190, 2001

Newport DJ, Stowe ZN, Nemeroff CB: Parental depression: animal models of an adverse life event. Am J Psychiatry 159:1265–1283, 2002

Newton ER: Breastmilk: the gold standard. Clin Obstet Gynecol 47:632–642, 2004

Nichols-Johnson V: Promoting breastfeeding as an obstetrician/gynecologist. Clin Obstet Gynecol 47:624–631, 2004

Niebyl JR, Blake DA, Freeman JM, et al: Carbamazepine levels in pregnancy and lactation. Obstet Gynecol 53:139–140, 1979

Nonacs R, Cohen LS: Assessment and treatment of depression during pregnancy: an update. Psychiatr Clin North Am 26:547–562, 2003

Nordeng H, Bergsholm YK, Bohler E, et al: The transfer of selective serotonin uptake inhibitors to human milk (in Norwegian). Tidsskr Nor Laegeforen 121:199–203, 2001

Ohman I, Vitols S, Tomson T: Lamotrigine in pregnancy: pharmacokinetics during delivery, in the neonate, and during lactation. Epilepsia 41:709–713, 2000

Ohman I, Vitols S, Luef G, et al: Topiramate kinetics during delivery, lactation, and in the neonate: preliminary observations. Epilepsia 43: 1157–1160, 2002

Ohman R, Hagg S, Carleborg L, et al: Excretion of paroxetine into breast milk. J Clin Psychiatry 60:519–523, 1999

Owens MJ, Morgan WN, Plott SJ, et al: Neurotransmitter receptor and transporter binding profile of antidepressants and their metabolites. J Pharmacol Exp Ther 283:1305–1322, 1997

Philbert A, Pedersen B, Dam M: Concentration of valproate during pregnancy, in the newborn and in breast milk. Acta Neurol Scand 72:460–463, 1985

Piontek CM, Baab S, Peindl KS, et al: Serum valproate levels in 6 breast-feeding mother-infant pairs. J Clin Psychiatry 61:170–172, 2000

Piontek CM, Wisner KL, Perel JM, et al: Serum fluvoxamine levels in breastfed infants. J Clin Psychiatry 62:111–113, 2001

Pynnonen S, Sillanpaa M: Carbamazepine and mother's milk (letter). Lancet 2(7934):563, 1975

Pynnonen S, Kanto J, Sillanpaa M, et al: Carbamazepine: placental transport, tissue concentrations in foetus and newborn, and level in milk. Acta Pharmacol Toxicol (Copenh) 41:244–253, 1977

Ragan KA, Stowe ZN, Brennan P, et al: The impact of maternal emotional well-being on infants. Poster presented at the 156th annual meeting of the American Psychiatric Association, San Francisco, CA, May 17–22, 2003

Rambeck B, Kurlemann G, Stodieck SR, et al: Concentrations of lamotrigine in a mother on lamotrigine treatment and her newborn child. Eur J Clin Pharmacol 51:481–484, 1997

Rampono J, Kristensen JH, Hackett LP, et al: Citalopram and demethylcitalopram in human milk; distribution, excretion and effects in breast fed infants. Br J Clin Pharmacol 50:263–268, 2000

Ratnayake T, Libretto SE: No complications with risperidone treatment before and throughout pregnancy and during the nursing period. J Clin Psychiatry 63:76–77, 2002

Ryan AS, Wenjun Z, Acosta A: Breastfeeding continues to increase into the new millennium. Pediatrics 110:1103–1109, 2002

Schimmell MS, Katz EZ, Shaag Y, et al: Toxic neonatal effects following maternal clomipramine therapy. J Clin Toxicol Clin Toxicol 29:479–484, 1991

Schmidt K, Olesen OV, Jensen PN: Citalopram and breast-feeding: serum concentration and side effects in the infant. Biol Psychiatry 47:164–165, 2000

Schou M, Amdisen A: Lithium and pregnancy, 3: lithium ingestion by children breast-fed by women on lithium treatment. Br Med J 2(5859): 138, 1973

Skausig OB, Schou M: Breast feeding during lithium therapy (in Danish). Ugeskr Laeger 139:400–401, 1977

Spencer JP, Gonzalez LS, Barnhart DJ: Medications in the breast-feeding mother. Am Fam Physician 64:119–126, 2001

Spigset O, Carieborg L, Ohman R, et al: Excretion of citalopram in breast milk. Br J Clin Pharmacol 44:295–298, 1997

Stahl MM, Neiderud J, Vinge E: Thrombocytopenic purpura and anemia in a breast-fed infant whose mother was treated with valproic acid. J Pediatr 130:1001–1003, 1997

Stewart R, Karas B, Springer P: Haloperidol excretion in human milk. Am J Psychiatry 137:849–850, 1980

Stowe ZN, Owens MJ, Landry JC, et al: Sertraline and desmethylsertraline in human breast milk and nursing infants. Am J Psychiatry 154: 1255–1260, 1997

Stowe ZN, Cohen LS, Hostetter A, et al: Paroxetine in human breast milk and nursing infants. Am J Psychiatry 157:185–189, 2000

Stowe ZN, Calhoun K, Ramsey C, et al: Mood disorders in pregnancy and lactation: defining issues of exposure and treatment. CNS Spectr 6:150–166, 2001

Stowe ZN, Hostetter A, Owens MJ, et al: The pharmacokinetics of sertraline excretion into human breast milk: determinants of infant serum concentrations. J Clin Psychiatry 64:73–80, 2003

Suri R, Stowe ZN, Hendrick V, et al: Estimates of nursing infant daily dose of fluoxetine through breast milk. Biol Psychiatry 52:446–451, 2002

Sykes PA, Quarrie J, Alexander FW: Lithium carbonate and breast-feeding. Br Med J 2(6047):1299, 1976

Taddio A, Ito S, Koren G: Excretion of fluoxetine and its metabolite, norfluoxetine, in human breast milk. J Clin Pharmacol 36:42–47, 1996

Tomson T, Ohman I, Vitols S: Lamotrigine in pregnancy and lactation: a case report. Epilepsia 38:1039–1041, 1997

Tsuru N, Maeda T, Tsuruoka M: Three cases of delivery under sodium valproate—placental transfer, milk transfer and probable teratogenicity of sodium valproate. Jpn J Psychiatry Neurol 42:89–96, 1988

Tunnessen WW Jr, Hertz CG: Toxic effects of lithium in newborn infants: a commentary. J Pediatr 81:804–807, 1972

Van den Bergh BR, Marcoen A: High antenatal maternal anxiety is related to ADHD symptoms, externalizing problems, and anxiety in 8- and 9-year olds. Child Dev 75:1086–1097, 2004

Verbeeck RK, Ross SG, McKenna EA: Excretion of trazodone in breast milk. Br J Clin Pharmacol 22:367–370, 1986

von Unruh GE, Froescher W, Hoffmann F, et al: Valproic acid in breast milk: how much is really there? Ther Drug Monit 6:272–276, 1984

Weinstein MR, Goldfield M: Lithium carbonate treatment during pregnancy; report of a case. Dis Nerv Syst 30:828–832, 1969

Weissman AM, Levy BT, Hartz AJ, et al: Pooled analysis of antidepressant levels in lactating mothers, breast milk, and nursing infants. Am J Psychiatry 161:1066–1078, 2004

Weissman MM, Prusoff BA, Gammon GD, et al: Psychopathology in the children (ages 6–18) of depressed and normal parents. J Am Acad Child Psychiatry 23:78–84, 1984

Whalley LJ, Blain PG, Prime JK: Haloperidol secreted in breast milk. Br Med J (Clin Res Ed) 282:1746–1747, 1981

Wilson JT, Brown RD, Cherek DR, et al: Drug excretion in human breast milk: principles, pharmacokinetics and projected consequences. Clin Pharmacokinet 5:1–66, 1980

Wisner KL, Perel JM: Serum nortriptyline levels in nursing mothers and their infants. Am J Psychiatry 148:1234–1236, 1991

Wisner KL, Perel JM: Nortriptyline treatment of breast-feeding women (letter). Am J Psychiatry 153:295, 1996

Wisner KL, Perel JM: Serum levels of valproate and carbamazepine in breastfeeding mother-infant pairs. J Clin Psychopharmacol 18:167–169, 1998

Wisner KL, Perel JM, Foglia JP: Serum clomipramine and metabolite levels in four nursing mother-infant pairs. J Clin Psychiatry 56:17–20, 1995

Wisner KL, Perel JM, Findling RL, et al: Nortriptyline and its hydroxymetabolites in breast-feeding mothers and newborns. Psychopharmacol Bull 33:249–251, 1997

Wisner KL, Perel JM, Blumer J: Serum sertraline and N-desmethylsertraline levels in breast-feeding mother-infant pairs. Am J Psychiatry 155:690–692, 1998

Woody JN, London WL, Wilbanks GD: Lithium toxicity in a newborn. Pediatrics 47:94–96, 1971

Yapp P, Ilett KF, Kristensen JH, et al: Drowsiness and poor feeding in a breast-fed infant: association with nefazodone and its metabolites. Ann Pharmacother 34:1269–1272, 2000

Yoshida K, Smith B, Craggs M, et al: Investigation of pharmacokinetics and of possible adverse effects in infants exposed to tricyclic antidepressants in breast-milk. J Affect Disord 43:225–237, 1997a

Yoshida K, Smith B, Kumar RC: Fluvoxamine in breast-milk and infant development (letter). Br J Clin Pharmacol 44:210–211, 1997b

Yoshida K, Smith B, Craggs M, et al: Fluoxetine in breast-milk and developmental outcome of breast-fed infants. Br J Psychiatry 172:175–178, 1998a

Yoshida K, Smith B, Craggs M, et al: Neuroleptic drugs in breast-milk: a study of pharmacokinetics and of possible adverse effects in breast-fed infants. Psychol Med 28:81–91, 1998b

Index

*Page numbers printed in **boldface** type refer to tables or figures.*